*Principles of Pediatric Fluid Therapy*

# Principles of Pediatric Fluid Therapy

Second Edition

## Robert W. Winters, M.D.

*Medical Director, Home Nutritional Support, Inc., Fairfield, New Jersey; formerly of the Department of Pediatrics, Columbia University College of Physicians and Surgeons, Columbia-Presbyterian Medical Center, New York*

*Little, Brown and Company*
*Boston*

# Contents

# Preface

Students, house officers, and practitioners have long expressed a need for a small book clearly delineating the relationships between theory and practice of fundamental physiologic principles of fluid therapy.

More than a decade ago Abbott Laboratories of North Chicago asked me to write such a primer. The result was a booklet of 100 pages, which Abbott distributed to thousands of students, house officers, and practicing physicians.

Those who care for pediatric patients are the booklet's primary audience. Pediatricians need a unifying approach that covers the entire range of size of patients that they are called on to manage. This book presents such a unifying, comprehensive set of clinically useful diagnostic and therapeutic principles that are equally applicable to all patients, large or small. I hope that future surgeons and internists as well as pediatricians will benefit by understanding the physiologic approach presented here. If one can master the problems of electrolyte and acid-base disorders in a pediatric setting, the basic information is easily transferred to a comparable adult setting.

The favorable reception of the first edition was mainly due to the small number of pages needed to present all the basic physiologic principles clearly and to show their practical applications. Experienced authors have long recognized that it is far more difficult to write a short book than a long one, and I can not only confirm this premise but can also add the corollary that the revision of a short book presents even greater challenges. The need to add new information competes with the need to maintain brevity. As a result the present book is necessarily longer than the first. I have expanded some areas, added information in response to questions raised by students, and related a few specific anecdotes from nearly three decades of work in this field. Finally, certain fundamental, as yet unanswered, questions are raised and discussed. Since these cannot be answered by hard information, I have formulated answers based on personal opinions. These opinions are clearly indicated as such, and I hope they will stimulate readers to challenge my views with well-designed studies that will result in sounder information.

For help rewriting this book, I wish to thank the Josiah Macy, Jr. Foundation for designating me a Faculty Scholar during a sabbatical leave in 1977. During that year, this revision was one of several projects. Thanks are due the London Hospital Medical College for appointing me an Honorary Professor of Physiology during that year. Special thanks are owed to Professor Kenneth Cross, Chairman of the Department of Physiology at the "London," in granting me total freedom of activity during this year, while at the same time standing ready to help at all times. The Commonwealth Fund provided a generous grant to defray library, typing, and illustration costs for the present revision as well as for other writing projects, and their support is gratefully acknowledged.

Finally, Fred Belliveau of Little, Brown and Company has been a constant source of encouragement. When I returned from sabbatical, two-thirds of the planned revisions had been through multiple drafts, but other parts of the book needed work, and the entire manuscript needed final polishing. These chores would have been completed in the ensuing year had not surgery and a protracted convalescence intervened. Only after returning to full-time academic duties and disposing of the mass of accumulated problems was a return to the task of completing the revision possible. Throughout this experience, Mr. Belliveau offered timely encouragement and support. Without it the revision might never have been finished.

R.W.W.

# I. Theory

Obligatory Loss     (ie) " maintenance $Rx$"

3-4 mea NaCl / kg / 24
2 meq $K^+$ / kg / 24

100cc/kg/24hr    0-10Kg
50cc / kg / 24hr    10-20
25cc / kg / 24     720

or 4cc - 2cc - 1cc / kg/hr

# 1. Disorders of Hydration

Disorders of hydration, acid-base equilibrium, or both are more commonly encountered in pediatric patients and often to a much more serious extent than in adult patients. There are several reasons why the infant and, to a lesser extent, the child are susceptible to these disorders. First, and most important, the normal rate of turnover per unit of body weight of water, electrolyte, acid, and base, as well as foodstuffs in infants is about three times that of the adult. Thus, any process that precludes the normal oral intake of food or fluid (e.g., vomiting) will deplete the body stores of water, electrolyte, acid, and base, as well as calories and protein (when expressed as percent of body weight) at much faster rates in infants and children than in adults. Second, the infant is more susceptible than the adult to the development of a number of disorders that produce abnormal losses of body water, electrolyte, acid, and base, the relative magnitudes of which far outstrip those of the adult with similar disorders. For example, infantile diarrhea can readily lead to losses of fluid in amounts up to 50 ml or more per kilogram of body weight in a single day; whereas, fluid loss due to diarrhea in an adult is rarely so large proportionately. Third, the infant's renal function, especially in the first few months, may not be as well developed as that of the adult and may be less able to counter or correct disorders of hydration and acid-base equilibrium. Therefore, it is hardly surprising that major problems of hydration, acid-base status, and nutrition constitute an important segment of the hospital practice of pediatrics. To formulate the therapy for such disorders requires a firm understanding of the underlying physiologic principles that govern the regulation of body water, electrolytes, and acid-base status, as well as an appreciation of the interaction of nutrition with these factors and with the process of growth.

## CHEMICAL ANATOMY OF THE BODY FLUIDS
### Total body water
The total body weight of any patient can be divided into a fraction that is water (total body water, TBW) and another fraction that is composed of solids; the latter consists of cell solids (largely pro-

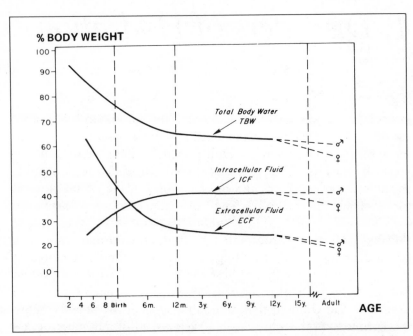

FIGURE 1. General patterns of change in total body water and its major subdivisions with prenatal and postnatal age. Note that the immediate postnatal changes (*see text*) are not shown.

tein), skeletal minerals, and body fat. A variety of techniques, generally involving either cadaver analysis or, more frequently, the measurement of the distribution of isotopic or non-isotopic tracer materials, have been applied to determine the normal or usual values for TBW in human subjects at various ages. Figure 1 shows the general trends observed in the proportion of the body weight that is water in normal individuals at various ages. In early prenatal life, body water per unit of body weight is very high; as gestation proceeds, body solids (i.e., protein, skeletal minerals, and depot fat) are increasingly deposited; hence, there is a progressive fall in the amount of TBW per unit of body weight. Thus, at term, the newborn infant has an average TBW of about 70 to 75 percent of body weight. In the early postnatal period, there is usually an abrupt loss of body water, amounting to 5 percent or more of the birth weight in the term infant. This loss of TBW, which is regarded as "physiologic," occurs while the infant is adjusting to the postnatal environment and establishing a completely satisfactory oral intake. After this initial adjustment, TBW averages about 65 percent of the body weight, a value that remains virtually

*[handwritten margin note:]* newborn TBW ,70.75(wt)]

*[handwritten margin note:]* TBW =65% wt

constant during the remainder of infancy and childhood. This constancy signifies that the increase in body fat and body solids is occurring proportionately to the increase in TBW.

At adolescence, characteristic sex differences in body composition occur. The normal, sexually mature adult male develops a greater muscle mass and less body fat than does the normal, sexually mature female. Because of these differences in body fat, the TBW of the adult male averages about 60 percent of the body weight; whereas, the TBW of the adult female, because of her normally greater amount of body fat, is less, averaging about 55 percent of the body weight.

### Subdivisions of the total body water

Traditionally, the total body water is divided into two major subdivisions—that portion of water present within cell membranes (*intracellular fluid*, ICF) and all water of the body that is excluded from cells (*extracellular fluid*, ECF). The ECF, in turn, is subdivided into two unequal compartments—the *plasma volume* (PV) and the *interstitial fluid* (ISF). A diagrammatic view of these subdivisions of the TBW is shown in Figure 2.

Much more elaborate models of the subdivisions of the TBW have been developed, including one that recognizes another major compartment, the *transcellular water*. Transcellular water is composed of all collections of fluid (e.g., cerebrospinal fluid, CSF) that have achieved a specific location by virtue of some transport process through specialized cells or tissues. In other words, it comprises the total secretory fluids of the body. Although these more complex models are useful for some purposes, for present purposes the simpler model shown in Figure 2 is adequate.

Changes in ECF as a function of age are shown in Figure 1 and can be compared to the patterns observed in TBW. In prenatal life, the higher TBW is associated with a proportionately higher value for ECF, and both of these compartments fall as growth of the fetus progresses during gestation, so that at term the ECF is about 35 to 40 percent of the body weight, and TBW is about 70 to 75 percent of the body weight. Blood volume is also relatively high at birth, owing principally to the higher packed-cell volume of the newborn infant. The fall in TBW noted in the immediate postnatal period comes about largely because of a commensurate fall in the ECF. Thereafter, ECF assumes a value of about 25 percent of the total body weight, a figure that remains fairly constant throughout normal infancy and childhood. After the characteristic adolescent

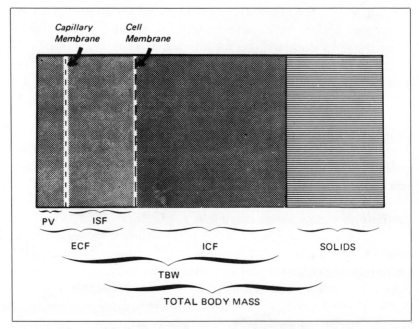

FIGURE 2. The total body mass and its major subdivisions into body solids and total body water (TBW). The latter is in turn subdivided into intracellular (ICF) and extracellular (ECF) compartments by the cell membrane. The ECF is in turn subdivided into interstitial fluid (ISF) and the plasma volume (PV) compartments by the capillary membrane.

changes in body composition occur, ECF values of about 20 percent are found in the normal adult male; somewhat smaller values are characteristic of the adult female.

Knowing the values for TBW and ECF permits the calculation of ICF since TBW = ECF + ICF. Values for ICF are also shown in Figure 1 and demonstrate that this compartment remains essentially constant in healthy subjects throughout life. Thus, the normal, age-dependent variations occurring in the TBW are almost entirely attributable to variations in the ECF; whereas, the age-conditioned variations in TBW are almost entirely attributable to changes in body fat (since body fat and TBW are inversely related to each other).

*Electrolyte composition of ECF and ICF*
The electrolyte compositions of the two major compartments of the TBW differ markedly from each other. These are diagrammed in Figure 3. The electrolyte composition of the ECF can be pre-

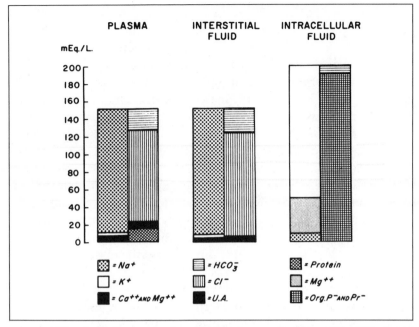

FIGURE 3. The electrolyte composition of the plasma, the ISF, and the ICF plotted on a "Gamblegram" where the cations (in mEq/L) are plotted cumulatively in the left column, and the anions are plotted in the right column. Because of the law of electroneutrality, the sum of the mEq/L of cations must equal the sum of the anions.

cisely determined because the plasma, a subcompartment of the ECF, is directly available for analysis. Figure 3 shows average normal values for plasma electrolytes plotted so that the column on the left represents the *cations* (positively charged ions) of the plasma—consisting of $Na^+$, $K^+$, $Ca^{++}$ and $Mg^{++}$—plotted as milliequivalents per liter (mEq/L). Since the law of electroneutrality must hold, the total height of the cation column must equal the total height of the *anion* (negatively charged ions) column on the right. The principal anions of plasma are chloride, bicarbonate, and protein. The difference in the negative charge of these three and the total is usually called the *undetermined anion* (UA) fraction, and it includes individual small contributions from inorganic sulfate and inorganic phosphate, as well as a number of organic acids, such as lactate, ketone bodies, and others.

anion gap

The electrolyte composition of the ISF can readily be derived from the plasma composition because the capillary membrane, which separates the ISF from the plasma, permits the free passage of water and all small ions and molecules but restricts protein (which has a negative charge) almost entirely to the plasma compartment. Thus, the concentrations of the cations in the ISF are virtually the same as in plasma (except for calcium, approximately half of which is bound to protein and therefore does not pass the capillary membrane). The anion pattern is similar, except for the lack of protein. However, the lack of negative charge owing to this lack of protein is made up by corresponding increases in the concentrations of the diffusible anions $Cl^-$, $HCO_3^-$, and undetermined anions, according to the principles of the Gibbs-Donnan equilibrium. In general terms, then, the ISF, which is the fluid to which the tissue cells are directly exposed, is nearly identical to the plasma in composition with the exception of the lack of protein. Furthermore, any change in the electrolyte composition of the ISF will be promptly reflected by similar changes in the plasma and vice versa. This aspect is important because the plasma is the only compartment of the body fluids that is directly accessible to the environment for sampling and intake.

Whereas the composition of the ECF can be estimated with great accuracy, the composition of the ICF can be only roughly approximated: tissue fluids, as such, cannot be obtained for accurate quantitative analyses. Furthermore, the ICF is a very heterogeneous compartment since it includes all cells of all tissues. Despite these limitations, much has been learned concerning cellular electrolytes, and from this information a general picture can be reconstructed (see Figure 3).

Compared to the ISF, which is basically a modified seawater containing large amounts of sodium and chloride and appreciable amounts of bicarbonate, the ICF generally contains little sodium, probably only tiny amounts of chloride, and relatively small amounts of bicarbonate. Instead, the major cations of the ICF consist principally of proteinates ($Pr^-$), organic phosphates ($OrgP^-$), and probably other as yet unidentified substances.

*Normal values for ECF electrolyte concentrations*
Normal adults have a remarkably constant sodium concentration in their plasma, averaging about 140 mEq/L with a range of about 137 to 143 mEq/L ($\pm$ about 2%). The normal plasma potassium averages about 4.0 mEq/L, with a range of about 3.8 to 4.5 mEq/L. The normal calcium concentration of the plasma is 10 mg/100ml, corresponding to 5 mEq/L, while the normal magnesium

concentration is about 2.0 mEq/L.* The total of all cations there-fore averages about 151 mEq/L, and the normal value for bicar-bonate is about 24 mEq/L. In venous plasma, bicarbonate concen-tration is higher by several milliequivalents per liter, because $CO_2$ is added by the tissues. The higher bicarbonate concentration in venous plasma is to a large extent offset by a lower concentration of chloride due to the "chloride shift" that occurs between eryth-rocytes and plasma when $CO_2$ is added to blood. The valence con-tributed by protein depends on the protein concentration, its dis-tribution between albumin and globulin, and the pH of the blood. If all these factors are normal, protein (more properly, proteinate) accounts for about 15 mEq/L of negative charge. Thus, from these three figures, we can compute the UA of the plasma:

$$UA = \text{total cation} - (Cl^- + HCO_3^- + Pr^-)$$
$$UA = 151 - (103 + 24 + 15) = 151 - 142 = 9 \text{ mEq/L}$$

As mentioned earlier, the UA consists of inorganic phosphate (about 2 mEq/L), inorganic sulfate (about 1 mEq/L), and organic and other anions (about 6 mEq/L).

The pattern of electrolytes in the plasma of infants closely re-sembles that of the adult, although there are certain quantitative differences. Infants have the same mean sodium concentration as do adults, although the range of normal may be slightly greater in infants, perhaps owing to the larger error introduced by micro-analysis. The plasma potassium also tends to be somewhat higher (but probably does not exceed about 5.0 mEq/L); again, sampling problems may be responsible for the larger, apparently normal variation of plasma potassium. Plasma calcium and magnesium concentrations in infants tend to be similar to those in normal adults.

The most notable differences between infant plasma and adult plasma concern the anions. The infant's arterial plasma bicarbon-ate concentration is distinctly less than that of the adult, having a value of about 20 mEq/L compared to 24 mEq/L in the adult. This reduction in bicarbonate concentration is offset by an increase in chloride concentration, with an average value being about 105 mEq/L and a slight increase in the undetermined anion. Of the latter, inorganic phosphate accounts for an additional 1 mEq/L or more, since the plasma inorganic phosphate in the growing infant

---

*See Glossary for definition of mEq and conversion of milligrams per 100 milliliters to milliequivalents per liter.

is higher than that in the fully grown adult. Total plasma protein concentration varies more in normal infants than in normal adults, and accordingly the valence contributed by protein is more variable; it averages approximately the same as or slightly less than the usual adult value.

In general, then, the infant plasma resembles the adult plasma, except for the lower bicarbonate and the slightly higher chloride and UA concentrations; a greater normal variation in the concentration of each of the electrolytes is, however, to be expected.

## OSMOMETRIC BEHAVIOR OF THE BODY FLUIDS*

### Fundamental considerations

The red cell is known to behave as a nearly perfect osmometer: When placed in a solution more concentrated than normal plasma, it shrinks; and when placed in a solution more dilute than normal plasma, it swells. These well-known changes in the erythrocyte are manifestations of the change in water content of the cell, with water leaving the cell and entering the medium in *hypertonic* solutions, and water entering the cell from the medium in *hypotonic* solutions. *Isotonic* solutions are those that cause no change in the size (and therefore in the water content) of the normal erythrocyte. Normal plasma is thus isotonic. Plasma containing a sodium concentration exceeding the normal 140 mEq/L would be hypertonic and would cause the erythrocyte to shrink; plasma containing a sodium concentration lower than normal would be hypotonic and would cause the erythrocyte to swell.

These changes in water movements across the erythrocyte cell membrane are manifestations of the fundamental phenomenon of *osmosis*. For an osmotic transfer of water to occur across any cell membrane, two conditions are required: (1) there must be a difference in the total concentration of non-permeating solutes on either side of the membrane, and (2) the membrane must be freely permeable to water. In the case of the erythrocyte (and most tissue cells), water permeates freely; whereas, the movement of sodium is regulated from within the cell by active metabolic processes that keep the concentration of sodium within the cell very low, which makes the membrane seem to be largely impermeable to sodium. Changing the external sodium concentrations thus causes predictable changes in water movement and, hence, in the volume of the

*See Glossary for definition of terms used in this section.

erythrocyte. Osmotic shifts of water are dependent strictly on the total number of solute particles present in the solution that do not penetrate the membrane. Such particles may be ions or undissociated molecules; they may be large or small; they may be positively or negatively charged, or they may have no charge at all. The essential requirement is that they be confined to the ECF.

In order to provide a uniform basis for the comparison of different types of solutions, the unit of *milliosmol* (mOsm) is used as a measure of the number of osmotic particles contributed by the solute to a solution. The definition of a mOsm can be formulated as follows:

mOsm = Millimols (mM) of substance × *n*

where *n* is the number of particles produced by dissociation of the substance. Thus, a 5% glucose solution contains about 280 mM of glucose per liter*, and *n* is 1 because glucose does not dissociate. Isotonic saline (0.85% NaCl) contains about 145 mM/L of NaCl and *n* is 2, since each mM of NaCl dissociates 1 mEq of $Na^+$ and 1 mEq of $Cl^-$. The mOsm/L for each of these solutions can be compared as follows:

For 5% glucose solution: 280 mM × 1 = 280 mOsm/L
For 0.85% saline solution: 145 mM × 2 = 290 mOsm/L

As is evident, these two solutions are similar in osmolarity (i.e., the mOsm/L), the differences being for the most part insignificant physiologically. For the most precise computation, account must be taken of the nonideal behavior of dissociable solutes by the use of a correction factor—the osmotic coefficient. This correction brings the osmolarity of these two solutions even closer to each other.

The osmolarity of the plasma can be deduced from its measured composition, which is depicted diagrammatically in Figure 4. When the osmotic contribution of each constituent of plasma is taken into account (and when corrected for nonideal behavior), the final value obtained is about 280 mOsm/L. Figure 4 clearly demonstrates that by far the most important contributors to the osmolarity of the plasma (and therefore to ISF) are sodium and its major accompanying anions, chloride and bicarbonate. Indeed, for nearly all practical purposes, the osmolarity of the plasma can

*A 5% solution contains 5 g/100ml = 50 gm/L or 50,000 mg/L; 180 mg is equivalent to 1 mM of glucose; therefore, mM/L of glucose = $\dfrac{50,000 \text{ mg/L}}{180 \text{mg/mM}}$ = 280 mM/L. See Glossary for definition of mM.

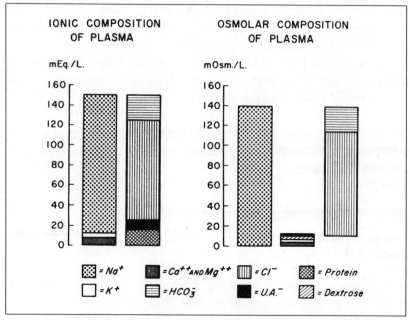

FIGURE 4. The osmotic contribution (in mOsm/L) of plasma electrolytes and non-electrolytes (glucose). Note that over 95% of the osmolarity of the plasma is accounted for by sodium and its accompanying univalent anions, chloride and bicarbonate.

be approximated simply by multiplying the sodium concentration of the plasma by 2:

$$\underset{\text{[mOsm/L]}}{\text{Plasma osmolarity}} = 2 \times \underset{\text{[mEq/L]}}{\text{plasma [ Na}^+]^*}$$

Since the normal plasma sodium is 140 mEq/L, the normal (isotonic) value for osmolarity is 280 mOsm/L.

## Osmometric behavior of the body water

Osmotic shifts of water between ECF and ICF are fundamental to an understanding of the internal redistribution of water that occurs in disorders of hydration. These are straightforward phenomena, since most tissue cells behave generally like the red cell with respect to these osmotic phenomena. Such osmotic behavior comes about primarily because sodium and its major anions, chlo-

---

*Throughout this book, square brackets [ ] will be used to designate concentrations of substances, whereas parentheses ( ) will be used to designate amounts of substances.

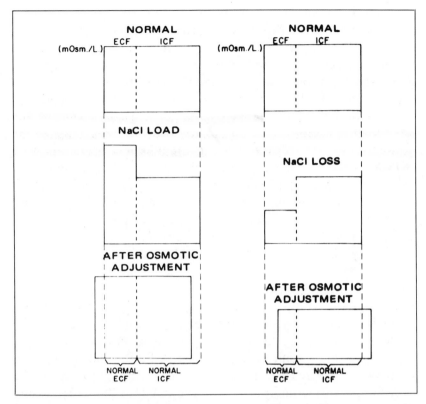

FIGURE 5. Internal redistribution of body water incident to gain or loss of NaCl without a change in content of total body water. The control (normal) diagram shows the volume of the TBW and its major subdivision on the horizontal axis. The vertical axis represents the osmolarity (i.e., 2 × plasma [Na⁺]). In each sequence, the intermediate step is a hypothetical one and shows the effect of gain or loss of NaCl in the ECF without any change in volume of ECF and before any shift in water has occurred. The last step shows the new final steady state after osmotic shifts of water have occurred.

ride and bicarbonate, are largely excluded from most tissue cells (see Figure 3); whereas, water permeates freely across all cell membranes. Thus, if one were to expose tissue cells to a hypertonic interstitial fluid, water would shift from the ICF to the ECF, causing tissue cell volume to shrink and extracellular fluid volume to expand commensurately. The opposite would happen if tissue cells were exposed to a hypotonic ISF.

Figure 5 depicts the steps involved in osmotic phenomena with changing ECF osmotic composition. The large rectangle represents the normal TBW with its two major subdivisions, ECF and ICF, separated from each other by the cell membrane, which excludes sodium and anions from cells but permits the free passage of water. The volumes of the compartments are shown on the horizontal axis, while the osmolarity is shown on the vertical axis— the normal value being 280 mOsm/L (i.e., 2 × normal plasma sodium concentration). Both ECF and ICF have the same osmolarity since water is free to move across the membrane. It is important to realize, however, that most of the osmolarity of the ECF is due to sodium, chloride, and bicarbonate ions; whereas, most of the osmolarity of the ICF is due to potassium, magnesium, and other intracellular ions. Hence, it is not the specific ionic or molecular species of each compartment but, rather, the sum of all nonpenetrating solutes, as expressed by the osmolarity, which determines the movement of water due to osmotic gradients.

Figure 5 shows the sequence of events that would occur if the osmolarity of the ECF were increased by adding sodium chloride without water. This type of abnormality could be produced by infusing a markedly hypertonic saline solution (e.g., 5% NaCl, which contains about 1700 mOsm/L) when the volume of the infusate is so small as to be negligible. If such an addition could be made instantaneously and the events "frozen" in a subsequent set of steps, the final result would be a marked difference in osmolarity between the two compartments. Given this gradient, in the next step, water would move from the ICF into the ECF, causing the former to shrink and the latter to expand, processes that are exactly analogous to suspending the erythrocyte in hypertonic media. The effect of this water movement is to reduce the ICF and to increase the ECF by exactly the same volume. A new steady state will be reached when the osmolarity of the two compartments is again equal. This new final osmolarity (and plasma sodium concentration) would be higher than normal but not as high as if the sodium chloride had been added to the ECF and no shift of water from the ICF had occurred.

The opposite result would be obtained if dry sodium chloride were removed from the ECF without a commensurate loss of water. This might occur if both solute and water were removed from the ECF and only the water replaced. Since only solute would have been removed (assuming that in the first step the volume of ECF would remain unchanged momentarily), osmolarity and plasma sodium concentration would fall. However, an osmotic gradient would now exist such that water would move into the ICF from the ECF until the osmolarity of the two phases were

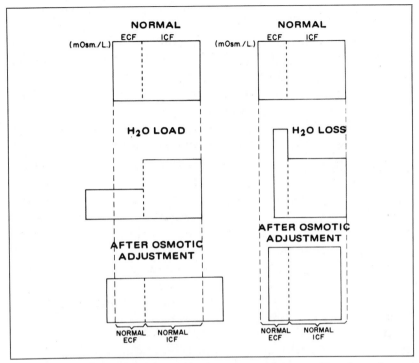

FIGURE 6. Internal redistribution of body water incident to gain or loss of water without a change in the content of body solute. The control (or normal) diagram shows the values of TBW, ECF, and ICF on the horizontal axis and the osmolarity of the body fluids (i.e., 2 × plasma [Na$^+$]) on the vertical axis. In each sequence, the intermediate step is a hypothetical one and shows the effect of gain or loss of water in the ECF without any change in the content of ECF solute. The last step shows the new final steady state after osmotic shifts of water have occurred.

again equal. The final result would be a decrease in ECF volume, an increase in ICF volume, and a fall in plasma sodium concentration in plasma osmolarity.

Thus far the "pure" effects of a gain or loss of sodium chloride without any change in TBW have been analyzed. There are two other "pure disturbances" that can be analyzed in exactly the same way—a gain of water and a loss of water without a change in the amount of total body solute (Figure 6). A pure gain of water initially would expand the ECF and dilute the extracellular solute so that ECF osmolarity and plasma sodium concentration would fall. A loss of water, on the other hand, would contract ECF volume, and, in the presence of the same amount of ECF solute, plasma osmolarity and plasma sodium concentration would rise. In each case, an osmotic gradient would be created, the result of which would be water movement to equalize the osmolarities of the two compartments. In the case of a gain of water, ICF would expand as ECF is contracted from its volumes prior to water transfer; in the final steady state, the volume of ECF would still be above the normal value, whereas its osmolarity and plasma sodium concentration would be reduced to below normal. In the case of water loss, ICF volume would be reduced, thus allowing a sharing of the ICF water in the total water loss; plasma osmolarity and plasma sodium concentration could rise.

The stepwise analyses in Figures 5 and 6 tend to obscure the fact that all movements of water between the ECF and ICF occur very rapidly. Therefore, one should never expect to find the pure changes depicted in the hypothetical intermediate steps in each of the four conditions depicted in these figures. Rather, the osmotic shifts of water begin immediately after any change in extracellular osmolarity and are largely complete within a matter of minutes. Thus, in evaluating a given value for sodium concentration in the plasma of a patient with a disorder of hydration, the clinician can safely assume that the osmotic transfer has already occurred and that a new steady state is present.

In all four examples shown in Figures 5 and 6, the route of loss or gain is via the ECF. This is because the ECF is the only compartment that communicates directly with the environment. Thus, the ECF—or more specifically the plasma, which is an integral part of the ECF—is in direct contact with the kidneys, the gastrointestinal tract, and the skin, and it is the only available route for any gain or loss to occur between the ICF and the environment. Any changes occurring in ICF volume or osmolarity are practically always secondary to changes in ECF volume and osmolarity.

One interesting situation of a *primary* increase occurring in intracellular osmolarity is during and just after a grand mal epileptic seizure. Apparently, when virtually the entire muscle mass is thrown into violent activity, "new" osmols, presumably intermediary metabolites, are produced in great numbers. These raise the osmolarity and the ICF, water moves into the ICF, and the ECF osmolarity and sodium concentration rise. This phenomenon is short lived but is an example of metabolic generation of idiogenic osmols.

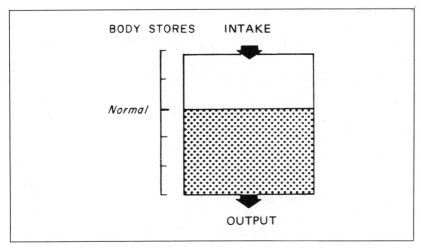

FIGURE 7. The balance principle as it may be applied to any substance (*X*)—e.g., water, Na⁺, Cl⁻, K⁺, and others. The amount of X of intake by *all* routes (represented by the arrow at the top) equals the amount of X lost by the body from *all* routes (represented by the arrow at the bottom). The balance of X is therefore zero, and the body stores of X, indicated by the scale at the side, remain constant (in this case at the normal level).

## EXTERNAL EXCHANGES OF WATER AND ELECTROLYTE WITH THE ENVIRONMENT

### The balance principle

In healthy persons the content of body water and body electrolyte is held remarkably constant from day to day despite considerable daily fluctuations of intake. Since intake of water and, especially, electrolytes do not appear to be closely regulated, this constancy implies the existence of finely tuned mechanisms regulating the renal output, which is mediated by antidiuretic hormone, aldosterone, and other factors capable of producing excretion of excesses of water and electrolyte intake or of conserving water and electrolyte when intake is restricted. It is useful to conceptualize such exchanges of water and electrolyte between the organism and the environment in terms of the *balance principle*. The balance principle simply states that the balance of any given substance in the body (X) is the difference between the intake of that substance by *all* routes and the output of that substance by *all* routes (Figure 7):

Balance of substance X = Intake of X − Output of X

It follows from this equation that the sign of the balance will reflect the directional change in the body stores of X. Thus, if the intake exceeds the output, the balance will be positive, and the body stores of X increase accordingly. If, on the other hand, the output of X exceeds the intake, the balance will be negative, and the body stores of X will fall. But if the intake of X equals the output of X, the body stores of X will remain constant at the preexisting level.

In the healthy, fully grown adult, the intake of water and electrolyte by all routes equals the output, so the balances of water and electrolyte over any appreciable period of time average zero; accordingly, the body stores remain constant at the normal level. In a growing infant, however, body stores increase because growth of new tissue requires deposition of new body water (both ICF and ECF), body potassium (in the ICF), and body sodium (in the ECF). When considered on a daily basis, however, these positive changes in the balance are very small. Furthermore, since growth ceases during illnesses that affect hydration or acid-base equilibrium, we can safely ignore the influence of growth on this component of the water balance over short periods of time as, for example, when an infant is receiving parenteral fluids for some illness.

The balance principle can also be applied to calories. To maintain caloric equilibrium—that is, a zero caloric or energy balance—an individual's net caloric intake must be equivalent to his total caloric expenditure, which consists of his basal expenditure plus added increments for specific dynamic action, physical activity, and other factors. Individuals who maintain a constant body composition are in zero external caloric balance. Individuals whose sustained caloric balance is positive gain weight since the excess calories are deposited in depot body fat; this is the only mechanism for disposing of excess calories. Individuals whose caloric intake is insufficient consume body fat to make up the energy difference. Normal, growing infants are always in positive caloric balance, since growth is associated with a proportional deposition of body fat as well as body water as part of the gain in total body weight. Furthermore, growth requires an energy expenditure for synthesis of new protein, and other functions. However, the additional intake of calories needed for growth is small compared to the total day-to-day intake and expenditure of calories; in ill infants and children we can disregard it altogether since unless a full dietary intake is provided, growth ceases entirely.

## Components of the intake

In healthy persons, the diet is the source of water intake, electrolyte, calories, and protein. Water includes not only the obvious fluids of the diet but also solid food, which is usually 60 to 80 percent or more water. Sodium, potassium, and chloride are, of course, present in food and may be augmented in the diet by the addition of salt in the preparation of food. In addition to dietary sources of water, there are two other "hidden" sources. One is the result of the normal oxidation of foodstuffs, particularly carbohydrate and fat:

$$\text{Carbohydrate or fat + oxygen} \longrightarrow CO_2 + H_2O$$

Such *water of oxidation* occurs whether the foodstuff oxidized is dietary or is of endogenous origin, as it is in the catabolism of body stores of carbohydrate or fat when caloric intake is inadequate. The second hidden source of water intake is the *preformed water* (water in the ICF) released into the ECF whenever there is tissue breakdown, such as in catabolic states or in wasting diseases. Similarly, the potassium in intact cells is a hidden source of intake that becomes available when the body tissue mass is catabolized or when there is destruction of necrotic tissue. Under most circumstances, these hidden sources of water or potassium are of little clinical significance. They become important, however, when there is severe impairment or complete absence of renal function, such as in the oliguric phase of acute tubular necrosis.

In addition to the components of intake, it is obvious that any parenteral administration of water or electrolyte must be counted as intake when both oral and parenteral fluids are provided. When the parenteral route is used exclusively, the quantities of water, sodium, potassium, chloride, and calories must be included as intake.

## Components of the output

Several components of the output of balance occur in health; others occur only in disease. In the healthy person, body water is lost through the skin, lungs, kidneys, and gastrointestinal tract. Normally, water evaporating through the skin and lungs serves to regulate temperature. Water lost in this fashion is called *insensible water loss* (IWL), so named because the individual does not sense its occurrence. IWL consists of pure water (i.e., without electrolyte).

Output
insensible - skin, lungs
sensible - sweat
stool (sm)
* urine

In addition to IWL, there is *sensible* water (and electrolyte) loss in the form of *sweat*. Sweating is a thermoregulatory mechanism, which unlike IWL is not continuous but rather is intermittent and dependent largely on the ambient temperature and the adequacy of other heat-losing mechanisms of the body. Sweat contains sodium and chloride as well as insignificant quantities of potassium. The average output of water owing to moderate sweating is approximately 30 to 40 mEq/L for both sodium and chloride ions, but there is considerable variation.

*Stool water losses* are ordinarily small in normal individuals passing formed stools. They can increase to very large proportions when diarrhea supervenes. This subject is discussed later, in the context of abnormal losses (see p. 19).

The *urine* is the principal route of water loss from the human organism. Unlike all the other routes discussed previously, the urine represents the only route of output that the body can control for the specific purpose of regulating body fluid volume and composition. In healthy persons, the kidney is the target of an abundant array of regulatory humoral and other mechanisms; these are capable of adjusting the urinary volume and the urinary excretion of electrolytes within broad limits to maintain optimal body stores of water, sodium, potassium, and chloride as well as an optimal acid-base status. In healthy persons, for example, the kidney excretes any excess of water and electrolyte not lost via the skin, lungs, or gastrointestinal tract, thereby maintaining a zero balance and constant body stores of these substances. The ability of the kidney to adjust to widely varying intakes or to extrarenal losses is remarkable. Large increases in the usual intake of water or electrolyte pose no serious problem to the balance of body fluids since the normal kidney accurately regulates urinary volume and composition and excretes the unwanted excess. Similarly, if the usual intake of water or electrolyte is moderately reduced in the face of the usual rates of extrarenal losses via the skin, lung, and gastrointestinal tract, urinary volume will be adjusted downward to maintain zero balance. Likewise, restriction of sodium or potassium intake is promptly reflected by reduced urinary excretion of these electrolytes so as to maintain nearly constant body stores. Of course, there are limits to both the degree of excess and the degree of restriction of either water or electrolyte to which the kidney can adjust. As for excess intake, the kidney has great tolerance, but such tolerance may be reduced by a variety of factors associated with disease. With restricted intake, the kidney suffers greater limitations. Thus, if water intake is zero, the kidney can at best produce minimal quantities of maximally concentrated urine and this will retard further losses of water from the body. But the kidney cannot make a water-free (solid) urine*, nor can it make "new" water available. Similarly, restriction of dietary sodium or potassium to zero levels will cause these electrolytes to virtually disappear from the urine; but if there are ongoing extrarenal losses of these substances, the kidney cannot make new sodium or potassium to replace them. Replacement can come only from exogenous or parenteral sources.

As has already been indicated, the ability of the kidney to adjust to wide variations of intake or to excesses or deficits of body stores may be limited by a host of factors in disease. The ability to concentrate urine may be impaired or the ability to excrete a large excess of water, sodium, or potassium may be limited. Likewise, the ability to maximally conserve sodium or potassium may be adversely influenced by illness or its treatment, such as stress, drugs, circulatory changes, reduction in glomerular filtration rate, and other factors. Furthermore, intrinsic renal disease itself may limit the maximally attainable renal function. All these factors must be considered in the formulation of reasonable water and electrolyte requirements for disease, a topic that will be discussed later. Figure 8 summarizes diagrammatically the components of intake and output for water in health, when a zero balance is achieved.

*Abnormal losses*

In addition to normal output that contributes to the balance of water and electrolyte, abnormal losses are encountered in many diseases. These may be classified as two general categories: (1) losses that occur through *normal* routes but in *abnormal amounts*, and (2) losses that occur through *abnormal* routes. Several commonly encountered examples in pediatric practice fall into the first category, the most notable of which are losses of water and electrolyte occurring via the gastrointestinal tract—for example, diarrhea. Diarrheal fluid consists essentially of modified small–intestinal juice that represents a mixture of glandular secretions of the small intestine, gastric juice, bile, pancreatic secretions, and partially digested food. Because of excessive motility of the gut and

---

*The maximal osmolarity achievable by the human kidney is about 1400 mOsm/L. Some desert rodents can produce urine at a concentration about 5 times greater than this, and such urine approaches a semisolid state.

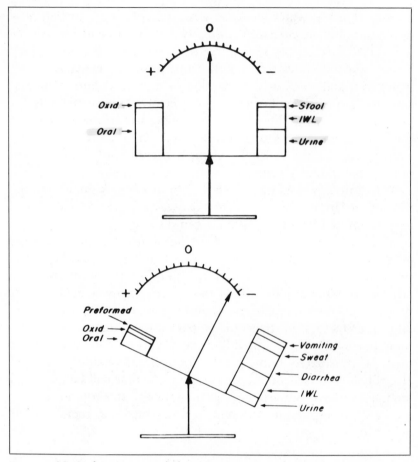

FIGURE 8. Normal (zero) water balance (top) compared with negative water balance as a result of diarrhea (bottom). The components of the intake are shown on the left side: dietary intake of water (in food and fluid) and water of oxidation. The components of the output are shown on the right side: insensitive water loss (IWL), sweat, stool water, and urine. The urine volume is the only component capable of adjustment to make output equal to intake.

other factors affecting the normal reabsorptive processes of the intestinal tract in diarrhea, the normal gastrointestinal fluids secreted initially to digest foodstuffs are lost from the body in a modified form. The stool electrolyte composition of infants with diarrhea is highly variable, but in general it is a hypotonic, multiple electrolyte-containing fluid. Average values approximate 40 mEq/L each of sodium, potassium, chloride, and bicarbonate, but the range of each of these is very wide. The volumes of such fluids that may be lost in moderate or severe diarrhea in an infant may

TABLE 1. Components of Balance of Water and Electrolyte During Development of Diarrheal Dehydration

| Intake of Water and Electrolytes | Output of Water and Electrolytes |
|---|---|
| Oral intake diminished owing to poor feeding and to vomiting | Insensible water loss continues at usual rate |
| | Sweating is probably present owing to ambient temperature conditions |
| | Urine is probably scant in volume; urinary excretion of $Na^+$ and $K^+$ is probably diminished to conserve diminished stores of these ions |
| | Diarrhea and vomiting occur with abnormal losses of water, $Na^+$, $K^+$, $HCO_3^-$, and $Cl^-$ |

be very large, reaching 5 percent or more (50 ml/kg) of the body weight of the patient in a given 24-hour period.

Another example of abnormal loss through a normal channel is in patients with cystic fibrosis; the sweat of these patients contains abnormally high concentrations of sodium and chloride (100 mEq/L or higher). This factor may cause no difficulty if the excessive loss is replaced by an adequate oral dietary intake, but if it is not replaced, salt depletion may ensue rapidly.

Abnormal losses may also occur through *abnormal channels*, the most important of which is loss of upper gastrointestinal secretions. Vomiting leads to losses of either hydrochloric acid (from the gastric juice), or losses of sodium, potassium, and bicarbonate (from upper intestinal secretions), or both. Fistula and/or tube drainage may likewise deplete the organism of water, sodium, potassium, and either hydrogen or bicarbonate ions, depending on the specific site of losses in the gastrointestinal tract.

In conceptualizing the balance of water or electrolyte in any given patient, *all* routes of gain and *all* routes of loss (both normal and abnormal) must be taken into account. Consider for example, an infant who develops diarrhea (see Figure 8). The pathogenesis of the dehydration, sodium depletion, and potassium depletion can be reconstructed in qualitative terms within the framework of the balance principle (Table 1). It is clear from this table that despite maximal renal conservation of water, sodium, and potassium (that may in themselves be seriously impaired by circulatory changes incident to dehydration), the infant will sustain large losses of body water, sodium, and potassium. These are likely to go unreplaced because of the inadequacy of oral intake offered or retained owing to the vomiting that so often accompanies diarrhea. In this setting, vomiting not only prevents adequate oral replacement but also produces further losses of water, sodium, and potassium. Hence, the negative water and electrolyte balances and their accompanying deficits of body stores come about through obvious losses of gastrointestinal secretions; these losses are augmented by further, less obvious losses of water and electrolyte through the skin, lungs, and urine in the face of an inadequate oral intake.

This analysis points logically to three general therapeutic aims in the management of such a patient: (1) attempt to stop any further loss (i.e., in this case, stop the diarrhea and vomiting, if possible), (2) assess the magnitude of water and electrolyte deficits, and restore them as rapidly and as safely as possible, and (3) provide enough water and electrolyte to meet ongoing losses while repair of the body water and electrolyte deficits is being carried out. A detailed approach to each of these facets of therapy is presented in Chapter 4.

# 2. Acid-Base Disorders

In healthy adults, the pH of blood is held within a very narrow range of about 7.38 to 7.42 (mean 7.40); whereas, in normal infants the mean value is the same (7.40), but the range is slightly greater, about 7.35 to 7.45. The extremes of blood pH compatible with life are difficult if not impossible to define since extreme distortions of blood pH are more likely to be a result than a direct cause of death. Nevertheless, in clinical medicine the extreme ranges of blood pH that may be encountered (and that are compatible with recovery) vary from 6.70 on the low side to 7.70 on the high side.

The ability of the organism to regulate the pH of blood within the narrow range of normal in health and to counter deviations of blood pH in disease basically involves the action of two distinct but closely interdigitated sets of mechanisms: (1) the physicochemical or buffer mechanisms that act as a first line of defense against excesses or losses of acid or base from the body fluids, and (2) the physiological mechanisms, principally involving the kidneys and the lungs, that act directly on the buffer mechanisms and make them much more efficient than would otherwise be the case.

## Buffer mechanisms

A *buffered solution* may be defined as one that contains a weak acid and its conjugate base. Such a solution is capable of minimizing pH changes when either acid or base is added, as compared to the pH of a solution with a comparable addition of acid or base to an equal volume of the same unbuffered solvent. The buffers in blood and in other compartments of the body fluids may be classified into two general groups: (1) the bicarbonate system, and (2) the nonbicarbonate system. In the former, carbonic acid ($H_2CO_3$) will for the moment be regarded as the weak acid (see the following equation) and bicarbonate ($HCO_3^-$), the conjugate base. In the case of the nonbicarbonate buffers, it is useful to treat all members of the group generically and use the symbols HBuf for the weak acid and Buf$^-$ for the conjugate base. In blood, the principal nonbicarbonate buffer is hemoglobin, with smaller contributions from inorganic and organic phosphate and plasma proteins. There is little if any nonbicarbonate buffer in the ISF, the principal buffer system in this compartment being the bicarbonate system. In the ICF, both groups are represented, with the nonbicarbonate buffers being composed of organic phosphate, proteins, and, probably, other substances.

The general operational characteristics of both classes of buffer systems, regardless of their location, is the same with respect to their responses to addition of strong acid or base. For example, *when a strong acid ($H^+X^-$) is added*, it is buffered by both classes of buffer such that the $H^+$ of the loading acid is largely converted to the weak acid members of the buffer pairs:

$$H^+X^- + B^+HCO_3^- \longrightarrow H_2CO_3 + B^+X^-$$
$$H^+X^- + B^+Buf^- \longrightarrow HBuf + B^+X^-$$

One way to visualize the effects of these buffers is to realize that they serve to diminish the free $H^+$ concentration of the solution by trapping the $H^+$ of the strong acid to produce the weak acids. Otherwise, a much larger concentration of free $H^+$ would have been produced by the strong tendency of dissociation of the strong acid. Weak acids have much lower tendencies for dissociation of free $H^+$. Thus, the resultant fall in pH, which is related inversely to the free $H^+$ of the solution, is minimized compared to that which would obtain if the same amount of $H^+X^-$ were added to an unbuffered solution.

*When a strong base is added ($B^+OH^-$)*, it is likewise buffered by both classes of buffers, such that the $OH^-$ of the strong base is converted to water by reaction with the weak acids of both classes of buffers:

$$B^+OH^- + H_2CO_3 \longrightarrow B^+HCO^- + H_2O$$
$$B^+OH^- + HBuf \longrightarrow B^+Buf^- + H_2O$$

Through these reactions, the degree of increase in pH that would have been produced by the addition of strong base to an unbuffered solution is minimized by trapping the $OH^-$ of the loading base to produce water, a substance in which the $OH^-$ has a much lesser tendency to dissociate.

The third buffer reaction of importance occurs whenever *carbonic acid or bicarbonate is gained or lost* by the system. Since a given buffer pair cannot buffer excesses or deficits of either member of the pair itself, the general buffer reaction occurring under these conditions involves an *interaction* between the members of the bicarbonate system and members of the nonbicarbonate system. The general form of this interaction equation is as follows:

$$H_2CO_3 + B^+Buf^- \rightleftharpoons B^+HCO_3^- + HBuf$$

Addition of the acid $H_2CO_3$ or loss of the base $HCO_3^-$ would tend to lower the pH, but this is ameliorated by the previous buffer reaction in the left-to-right direction. Conversely, loss of the acid $H_2CO_3$ or gain of the base $HCO_3$ tends to increase the pH, an effect minimized by the previous buffer reaction in the right-to-left direction.

All buffers of both the bicarbonate and nonbicarbonate systems in all body fluid compartments are in some type of equilibrium with each other; changes in one compartment are therefore reflected by changes in all of the other compartments. In the case of equilibrium between the erythrocyte and the plasma, the passage of the relevant reactants and products occurs by the process of diffusion, except for hemoglobin, an important nonbicarbonate buffer that, because of its size, is confined to the erythrocyte. The acid-base equilibria between the ECF and the ICF and between the ECF and bone almost certainly do not represent simple diffusion processes but, rather, involve much more complex mechanisms. Although these mechanisms are not known in great detail, it is certain that both bone and ICF nonbicarbonate buffers play a quantitatively important role in the response of the organism to acid-base disorders.

The recognition of these multiple equilibria is of practical importance since it means that acid-base phenomena can be analyzed, at least qualitatively, in terms of a single buffer system in the plasma, rather than having to take account of all buffer systems in all phases of the body fluids—a virtually insurmountable conceptual obstacle at this stage of our knowledge. The buffer system most commonly used to analyze acid-base phenomena is the bicarbonate-carbonic acid system in the plasma. This system has two advantages for this purpose: (1) it can be characterized by accurate quantitative laboratory methods, and (2) it is the direct target for physiological regulation by the lungs and the kidneys.

## The Henderson-Hasselbalch equation

In order to use the plasma bicarbonate buffer system for the clinical analysis of acid-base disturbances, it is necessary to quantitate the relationships between the weak acid (carbonic acid), the conjugate base (bicarbonate), and pH. These relationships are formalized by the well-known Henderson-Hasselbalch equation, which in its most general form, is as follows:

$$pH = pK' + \log \frac{[\text{conjugate base}]}{[\text{weak acid}]}$$

This equation simply states that blood pH is equal to a constant, pK', plus the logarithm of the concentration of the conjugate base over the concentration of the weak acid. Thus, pH varies not with the concentration of the numerator *alone* nor with the concentration of the denominator *alone* but rather with the *ratio* of the numerator to the denominator.

Applying this equation to the bicarbonate system in which $HCO_3^-$ is the base form and $H_2CO_3$ represents, for the moment, the weak acid form results in the following equation:

$$pH = pK' + \log \frac{[HCO_3^-]}{[H_2CO_3]}$$

The operational characteristics of the Henderson-Hasselbalch equation can be illustrated by substitution of mean values for normal arterial blood plasma. In arterial blood, the value for pK' is 6.10 and is a constant. The normal arterial plasma bicarbonate concentration in adults is about 24.0 mEq/L, whereas the normal denominator term has a value of 1.2 mM/L. Thus, the equation for normal arterial blood plasma can be solved for blood pH as follows:

$$\text{Blood pH} = 6.10 + \log \frac{24.0}{1.2}$$

$$\text{Blood pH} = 6.10 + \log \frac{20}{1}$$

Since the log of $^{20}/_1$ is 1.30, the equation reduces to

$$\text{Blood pH} = 6.10 + 1.30 = 7.40$$

Thus, substituting normal values gives the correct value for the normal mean arterial blood pH of 7.40. For normal infants, both numerator (20 mEq/L) and denominator (1.0 mM/L) are less than in adults, but the ratio (20 : 1) is the same and the normal pH is the same, 7.40:

$$\text{Blood pH} = 6.10 + \log \frac{20.0}{1.0} = 6.10 + 1.30 = 7.40$$

It should be noted that the Henderson-Hasselbalch equation contains three unknowns—the numerator term, the denominator term, and pH. This means that to solve the equation completely, two of the three unknowns must be measured and the third calculated. In current practice, pH and $PCO_2$ (related to the denominator term, as explained in the following section) are determined, and bicarbonate concentration is computed. An older method relied upon the determination of pH and the plasma total $CO_2$ content (the latter representing the sum of the numerator and the denominator), and with this information the equation could be solved as well.

### Nature of the denominator term

The denominator term in the Henderson-Hasselbalch equation has thus far been treated as carbonic acid without elaboration. In fact, the denominator term consists of two components: "true" carbonic acid ($H_2CO_3$) and dissolved $CO_2$ ($CO_{2(d)}$). This is because carbonic acid in aqueous solution always exists in equilibrium with dissolved $CO_2$ through the so-called hydration reaction.

The hydration reaction is catalyzed by the enzyme, carbonic anhydrase, which is present in abundance in the erythrocyte and in certain other tissues. The hydration reaction is as follows:

$$CO_{2(d)} + H_2O \rightleftharpoons H_2CO_3$$

The Henderson-Hasselbalch equation, when properly written to take account of the true nature of the denominator term, is as follows:

$$\text{Blood pH} = 6.10 + \log \frac{[HCO_3^-]}{[H_2CO_3] + [CO_{2(d)}]}$$

Recognition of this interrelationship between carbonic acid and dissolved $CO_2$ is important because blood in the pulmonary capillary comes into equilibrium with alveolar air that contains gaseous $CO_2$ (Figure 9). This equilibrium follows the simple gas law known as *Henry's law*, which in its most general form states that the amount of gas dissolved in a liquid is equal to the pressure of the particular gas in the gas phase multiplied by a specific solubility coefficient for that gas in that particular liquid. Thus, if the

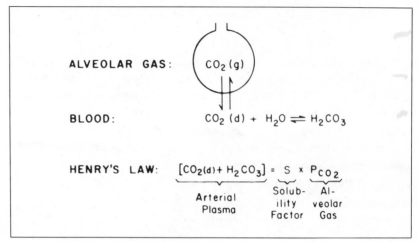

FIGURE 9. Relationship between $PCO_2$ of alveolar gas and the concentrations of $CO_{2(d)} + H_2CO_3$ in arterial plasma.

pressure of $CO_2$ in the gas phase is abbreviated as $PCO_2$ the amount of $CO_2$ dissolved in blood (plus that converted to carbonic acid, which cannot easily be separated from dissolved $CO_2$) is given by the following expression:

$$PCO_2 \times S = [CO_{2(d)} + H_2CO_3]$$

$S$ is the solubility factor for $CO_2$ in the blood, and at body temperature it is a constant having a value of 0.03 mM of gas dissolved per liter of plasma per mm Hg of $PCO_2$. Thus, using the normal adult value for $PCO_2$ of 40 mmHg along with the constant value of 0.03 for $S$ gives the following equation for normal conditions:

$$40 \text{mm Hg} \times 0.03 \text{ mM/L/mm Hg} = 1.2 \text{ mM/L}$$
$$(PCO_2) \times \qquad (S) \qquad = [CO_{2(d)} + H_2CO_3]$$

The value of 1.2 mM/L for the denominator term of course agrees with the value derived preceding for the normal arterial blood pH.

*Respiratory regulation of acid-base equilibrium*
The preceding considerations demonstrate an alternative way to write the Henderson-Hasselbalch Equation—by substituting $34S \times PCO_2$ for the term $H_2CO_3 + CO_{2(d)}$:

$$\text{Blood pH} = 6.10 + \log \frac{[\text{HCO}_3^-]}{[S \times \text{PCO}_2]}$$

For most clinical purposes, this is the form of the equation used since it emphasizes that it is the level of $PCO_2$ in the alveolar gas that determines the denominator term. In other words, clinical practice strongly favors the use of $PCO_2$ expressed in mm Hg rather than the more awkward term of $H_2CO_3 + CO_{2(d)}$ expressed in mM/L. So long as one understands the roles of the hydration reaction and Henry's law, this should lead to no confusion. This usage is certainly to be preferred to the use of $H_2CO_3$ alone as the denominator term, since this ignores the quantitatively important effect of the hydration reaction on the apparent strength of $H_2CO_3$ as an acid.

Actually, $H_2CO_3$ when studied in the absence of $CO_{2(d)}$ is a relatively strong acid, having a pK' of about 3.8. The equilibrium between $H_2CO_3$ and $CO_{2(d)}$ in the hydration reaction is such that there are about 800 parts $CO_{2(d)}$ for every part of $H_2CO_3$. The value of 6.1 for pK' in the Henderson-Hasselbalch equation takes account of this fact; hence, the only proper way of depicting the denominator term is $[H_2CO_3 + CO_{2(d)}]$.

Respiratory regulation of blood acid-base status occurs by regulation of $PCO_2$; this occurs by adjusting the rate of alveolar ventilation to reduce (with alveolar *hyperventilation*) or increase (with alveolar *hypoventilation*) alveolar $PCO_2$ as shown in Figure 10. For example, in healthy persons the $CO_2$ produced by the tissues is transported by the venous blood to the lungs and expelled. Alveolar ventilation is regulated by the respiratory center to keep alveolar $PCO_2$ at 40 mm Hg, a level at which the normal (adult) value of 1.2 mM/L for the denominator term is maintained in the arterial plasma. If $CO_2$ production remains constant, the doubling of alveolar ventilation reduces by one-half the $PCO_2$ (to 20 mm Hg); accordingly, the denominator falls to 0.6 mM/L. Halving alveolar ventilation causes $PCO_2$ to double (to 80 mm Hg), and with $CO_2$ production remaining constant, the value of the denominator term rises to 2.4 mM/L.

In *respiratory* disturbances of acid-base equilibrium, there is a primary abnormality at some level of the respiratory system (lung, respiratory musculature, neural connections, or peripheral or central regulation), and alveolar ventilation is altered to a higher or lower level than normal. A primary alveolar *hyperventilation* is

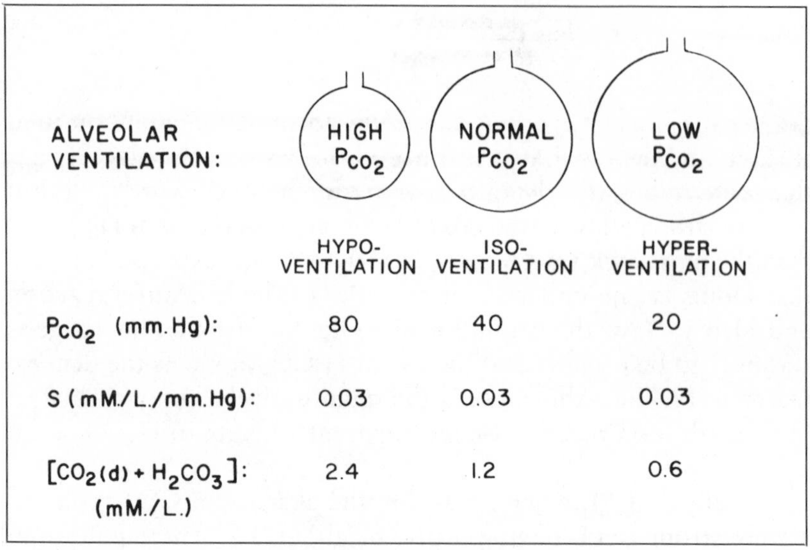

| ALVEOLAR VENTILATION: | HIGH $P_{CO_2}$ | NORMAL $P_{CO_2}$ | LOW $P_{CO_2}$ |
|---|---|---|---|
| | HYPO-VENTILATION | ISO-VENTILATION | HYPER-VENTILATION |
| $P_{CO_2}$ (mm.Hg): | 80 | 40 | 20 |
| S (mM./L./mm.Hg): | 0.03 | 0.03 | 0.03 |
| $[CO_{2(d)} + H_2CO_3]$: (mM./L.) | 2.4 | 1.2 | 0.6 |

FIGURE 10. Influence of a change in alveolar $PCO_2$ on the $[CO_{2(d)} + H_2CO_3]$ of arterial plasma.

the fundamental abnormality in *respiratory alkalosis*, and it causes a decrease in $PCO_2$ with a resulting decrease in the value of the denominator, an increase in the value of the ratio, and an alkaline shift in pH. The opposite disorder in alveolar ventilation leads to an increase in $PCO_2$ and *respiratory acidosis*.

In two other general types of acid-base disturbances, the so-called metabolic disturbances, the primary abnormality affects the metabolic component and is reflected by a rise or fall in plasma bicarbonate concentration. Hence, in *metabolic acidosis*, there is a gain of strong acid or a loss of bicarbonate, either of which results in a fall in the value of the numerator and a decrease in the value of the ratio and, hence, in pH. This lowering of pH in turn stimulates the respiratory center to produce a secondary alveolar *hyperventilation* and $PCO_2$; hence, the value of the denominator term decreases. This fall in $PCO_2$ ameliorates the acid shift in pH tending to restore it toward normal. This secondary physiologic response is known as *respiratory compensation* to metabolic acidosis.

The opposite occurs in *metabolic alkalosis*, in which the primary abnormality is an increase in the plasma bicarbonate concentration due to a gain of strong base or bicarbonate. Here the alkaline pH produced by the increase in the value of the ratio is ameliorated by a secondary increase in the value of the denomi-

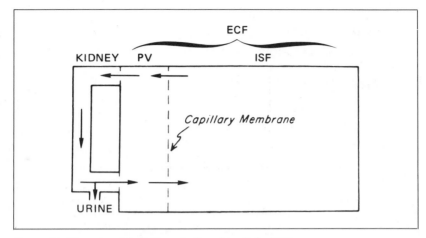

FIGURE 11. The role of the kidney in "washing" the ECF.

nator term. Alveolar *hypoventilation*, thus, is the expected *respiratory compensation* in metabolic alkalosis.

## Renal regulation of acid-base equilibrium

While the respiratory system is primarily responsible for the level of $PCO_2$ and, hence, value of the denominator term of the Henderson-Hasselbalch ratio, the kidney is responsible for the regulation of the bicarbonate concentration or the value of the numerator term. The detailed intrinsic mechanisms responsible for the renal control of bicarbonate concentration will not be dealt with here. Rather, it is sufficient for present purposes to regard the kidney as a "black box" through which flows a large amount of blood via the renal circulation and from which exits urine of varying acid-base composition depending on the needs of the organism. Thus, the urine provides a means for excretion of unwanted acid or base, thereby "cleansing" the renal arterial blood and returning that blood via the renal venous system to the general circulation; here, the blood exchanges bicarbonate directly with the entire ECF (Figure 11) and indirectly with the ICF and bone. In considering this role of the kidney, it is important to bear in mind that in any given 24-hour period, the renal blood flow is sufficiently large to process the entire ECF volume some 15 times. The kidney can therefore adjust a disturbed ECF acid-base equilibrium by producing rather rapidly a major upward or downward change in the bicarbonate concentration of the body fluid.

Basically, the kidney can perform two different operations affecting the bicarbonate concentration of the ECF, and it performs

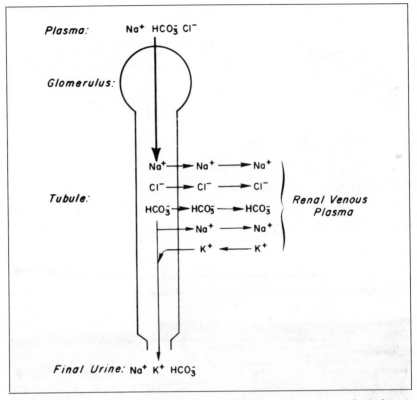

FIGURE 12. The overall role of the kidney in alkalinizing the urine. The kidney is depicted as a single nephron with a glomerulus and tubule. $Na^+$ and $HCO_3^-$ of the plasma are filtered at the glomerulus and enter the tubular urine where some is reabsorbed by the proximal tubule. The remaining fraction is delivered to the distal nephron where some of the $Na^+$ is reabsorbed in exchange for $K^+$, so that the final urine contains $HCO_3^-$ with a mixture of $Na^+$ and $K^+$.

one or the other according to the need for regulation or restoration of blood pH. In the first, bicarbonate entering the kidney in the renal arterial blood escapes into the environment (Figure 12). The result is the loss of bicarbonate from the ECF and a fall in bicarbonate concentration in the renal venous blood and, hence, in the ECF as a whole. The process of producing a bicarbonate-rich urine under such conditions is called *alkalinization of the urine.* This mechanism can be expected to operate in any situation in which there is either a relative excess of bicarbonate (as in acute respiratory alkalosis) or an absolute excess of bicarbonate (as in metabolic alkalosis). In the former case, the reduction of plasma bicarbonate concentration to an appropriate, abnormally low, value restores blood pH to normal in the face of a fixed, lowered value for $PCO_2$ because of the primary respiratory defect. Hence, this process is referred to as *renal compensation* to respiratory alkalosis. In metabolic alkalosis the plasma bicarbonate is supernormal, and the excretion of bicarbonate constitutes a *corrective measure* rather than a compensatory one, since in this case the primary disturbance—i.e., the supernormal level of plasma bicarbonate concentration—is being reduced toward normal.

It is important to point out that the ability of the kidney to alkalinize the urine requires that bicarbonate, an anion, be excreted along with a cation—either sodium or potassium, to satisfy the demands of electroneutrality. As long as there are no body sodium or potassium deficits or any other restrictions on the excretion of these cations, the kidney will excrete bicarbonate in an alkaline urine. But if body stores of these ions are depleted significantly or if there are other restrictions on the excretion of these ions imposed by disease (e.g., heart failure with avid sodium reabsorption), the cations will be conserved. A further complicating factor in limiting bicarbonate excretion is the presence of *hypochloremia*, which, of course, also accompanies an increase in plasma bicarbonate concentration. Given hypochloremia plus stimuli for cation conservation, bicarbonate excretion is severely limited. The result then is an acid and not an alkaline urine; this is known as the syndrome of *paradoxical aciduria with systemic alkalosis*. This seemingly anomalous response is a clue to the clinician to replenish sodium, potassium, and chloride stores. Correction of this situation obviously requires repletion of chloride stores given as the sodium or potassium salts.

The second possible operation of the kidney in bicarbonate regulation is the ability of the kidney to make "new" bicarbonate available to the ECF. This occurs when there is a relative decrease (respiratory acidosis) or absolute decrease (metabolic acidosis) in the plasma bicarbonate concentration so that blood pH is low. In metabolic acidosis (see the preceding text), plasma bicarbonate concentration is absolutely reduced, and despite respiratory compensation, blood pH is usually low. Under these conditions, the normal kidney often can produce a definitive *correction* by readjusting plasma bicarbonate to normal and, following a respiratory readjustment of $PCO_2$, the acid-base status of body fluids is completely restored to normal. In respiratory acidosis with a high fixed value for $PCO_2$, there is a relative deficit of plasma bicarbonate and blood pH is low. In this condition the kidney can produce a secondary rise in plasma bicarbonate concentration to supernor-

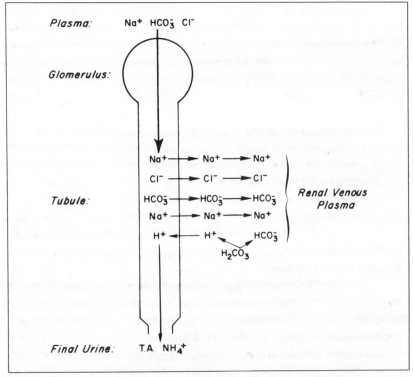

FIGURE 13. The overall role of the kidney in acidification of the urine. $Na^+$ and $HCO_3^-$ enter the glomerular filtrate, and the latter is entirely reabsorbed in the proximal tubule. Acidification occurs in the distal nephron. Note that for every $H^+$ excreted into the final urine (as TA or $NH_4^+$; see text), one "new" $HCO_3^-$ is made available to the plasma and, hence, to the ECF.

mal levels such that blood pH is raised to or toward normal. This constitutes *renal compensation* to the respiratory acidosis.

It is apparent from the foregoing that to achieve an elevation of the plasma bicarbonate concentration of the ECF in either metabolic or respiratory acidosis, the kidney must in essence produce new bicarbonate, and it does this by a process known as *acidification of the urine*. The overall mechanism is depicted in Figure 13. The renal tubular cell, starting with dissolved $CO_2$ and water, forms carbonic acid, then splits it into hydrogen ions and bicarbonate ions. The hydrogen ions are secreted into the tubular urine in exchange for sodium ions, which are reabsorbed from the tubular urine and returned to the peritubular plasma and, hence, to the ECF. The hydrogen ions secreted into the lumen are not excreted free in the final urine but rather appear in the urine in one of two buffered forms, *titratable acid* (TA) or *ammonium* ($NH_4^{++}$).

Urinary titratable acid is derived by the following equation:

$$HPO_4^{2-} \quad + \quad H^+ \quad \longrightarrow \quad H_2PO_4^-$$

*(tubular urine)*          *(from renal*        *(final urine)*
                          *tubular cell)*

Urinary ammonium is derived by the following overall equation:

$$Amino\ acids \longrightarrow NH_3 \quad + \quad H^+ \quad \longrightarrow \quad NH_4^+$$

                    *(from renal*        *(from renal*        *(final urine)*
                    *tubular cell)*       *tubular cell)*

The essential point about both these mechanisms is that "free" $H^+$ is bound so that large quantities of $H^+$ can be excreted in the final urine within the lower limit of the urine pH, which is about 4.50.

Thus, under conditions of metabolic acidosis or respiratory acidosis, the urine may be expected to contain large amounts of TA and $NH_4^+$ and have an acid pH, conditions that signify an augmented production of new bicarbonate by the kidney; the bicarbonate is returned to the renal venous blood and ultimately causes a rise in the bicarbonate concentration of the whole ECF.

The term *net acid excretion* (NAE) is often used to signify the net contribution of the kidney to the excretion of acid (or base). NAE is defined as the daily urinary TA + $NH_4^+$ − $HCO_3^-$ and can be determined readily by a titrimetric method on a 24-hour urine sample. It is obvious from the foregoing that for every mEq of NAE excreted in the urine, one mEq of "new" $HCO_3^-$ is returned to the renal venous plasma and, hence, to the body fluid. In alkaline urine, NAE is, of course, negative owing to the large excretion of $HCO_3^-$ and the minimal excretion of TA and $NH_4^+$. In passing, it is noteworthy that the urine pH discussed in the preceding text conveys very little information about the magnitude of urinary excretion of acid or base from the body. To estimate the latter requires that the NAE be determined.

Just as there are limitations on the kidney in alkalinizing the urine in alkalotic states, there are limitations on the kidney in acidifying the urine in acidotic states. This is particularly so when dehydration and salt depletion coexist with acidosis and it is probably owing to a combination of factors, such as reduced renal blood flow (which often accompanies dehydration) plus inadequate amounts of glomerular filtrate delivered to the distal portions of the nephron where the acidification mechanism is located. But even when these limitations are not present, the kidney's ability to acidify the urine is not unlimited. Furthermore, even under optimal conditions it takes at least several days for the normal kidney to achieve maximal rates of ammonium production, and it is the ammonium mechanism rather than the titratable acid mechanism that is quantitatively the most important means of excreting hydrogen ions into the environment.

In considering acid-base regulation, it is important to recognize that there is a distinct difference in the time needed for the respiratory mechanism to exert its effects on blood acid-base status as opposed to the renal mechanism. Thus the respiratory regulation of $PCO_2$ is evident in a matter of a few minutes, although full readjustment of the respiratory mechanism to achieve maximal sustained respiratory compensation in a metabolic acid-base disorder probably requires 12 hours or more. On the other hand, the kidney requires some hours to produce even a slight effect upon plasma bicarbonate concentration and several days or more to produce a sustained maximal effect sufficient to evoke a major change in the body buffers.

## SUMMARY OF PATHOPHYSIOLOGY OF ACID-BASE DISTURBANCES

### Terminology of acid-base disorders

In discussing acid-base abnormalities, it is important to respect the agreed upon terminological usage to avoid confusion and misunderstanding. *Acidosis* and *alkalosis* are generally defined as abnormal physiologic states; the modifying adjectives, *respiratory* and *metabolic*, signify general etiologies for these abnormal states. Although the observed analytical data on blood acid-base status (blood pH, plasma $PCO_2$, and plasma $HCO_3^-$ concentration) are preferably reported as the actual numerical data, there is often a need for words to describe the directional abnormalities observed in a given patient. The following are the usually accepted words for these purposes: *acidemia* and *alkalemia* for deviations in blood pH; *hypercapnia* (or hypercarbia), and *hypocapnia* (or hypocarbia) for deviations in $PCO_2$; *hyperbasemia* and *hypobasemia* for deviations in plasma bicarbonate.

Each acid-base disorder has a general etiology that produces a primary abnormality in either the metabolic or the respiratory component. *Compensation* refers to those secondary physiologic adjustments directed against the component *not* primarily affected, those components producing a change to restore pH toward normal. *Correction* of an acid-base disturbance, on the other hand, refers to the physiologic or therapeutic mechanisms directed at the component *primarily* affected by the etiologic factor, those producing a change to restore pH toward normal.

Tables 2 and 3 present the four so-called simple acid-base disorders in terms of the etiologic factors, the buffer mechanisms responsible, and the compositional changes expected in the plasma. Each of these will be discussed in turn.

*Metabolic acidosis*
All forms of metabolic acidosis can be classified into one of two general categories: (1) those produced by the gain of a strong acid by the ECF, and (2) those produced by the loss of bicarbonate from the ECF. In the first category, the acids commonly involved are the ketone bodies (β-hydroxybutyric and acetoacetic acids, as in diabetic acidosis, starvation ketoacidosis, and the acidosis of salicylate poisoning); phosphoric, sulfuric, and other acids (in azotemic renal failure); or lactic acid (occurring either secondary to tissue hypoxia due to poor perfusion or hypoxemia; or in the rare primary lactic acid acidosis). The second general cause of metabolic acidosis is bicarbonate loss. This can come about because of an abnormal loss of bicarbonate via the kidney (as in renal tubular acidosis) or because of a loss of an alkaline small-intestinal fluid. Thus, such disorders as diarrhea, drainage of small-intestinal fistulae, and suction of small-intestinal juices produce bicarbonate-losing metabolic acidosis.

The pH of diarrheal stools is usually acid, a finding that at first glance seems to contradict the idea that diarrhea is accompanied by a loss of bicarbonate. This paradox is readily explained when one realizes that the initially alkaline small-intestinal juices are further subjected to extensive bacterial fermentation, and organic acids are produced. These acids are neutralized by the bicarbonate-containing secretions in the gut; hence, pH falls to acid levels. Analysis of the final stool will show an *anion gap* (the difference between total cations and total anions; see Glossary) equal to the original bicarbonate content. Direct, detailed analysis will show the presence of organic acids of bacterial origin in abundance and equivalent to the anion gap. In cholera, where the transit time is extremely rapid, stool pH is usually alkaline due to insufficient time for the intermediate bacterial reactions.

The general buffer reactions in metabolic acidosis, shown in Table 2, lead to a primary fall in the bicarbonate concentration. Compensation is respiratory with a secondary lowering of plasma $PCO_2$.

TABLE 2. Etiologies and Compositional Changes in Plasma in Metabolic Acid-Base Disorders

| Disturbance | General Etiology | Clinical Examples | Buffer Reactions | Changes in Plasma | | |
|---|---|---|---|---|---|---|
| | | | | $[HCO_3^-]$* | $PCO_2$† | pH |
| Metabolic acidosis | Gain of strong acid by ECF | Ketone acids: diabetes, starvation, salicylism<br>Phosphoric and sulfuric acids: azotemic acidosis<br>Lactic acid: primary lactic acid acidosim tissue hypoxia | $H^+X^- + B^+HCO_3^- \longrightarrow$<br>$H_2CO_3 + B^+X^-$<br>$H^+X^- + B^+Buf^- \longrightarrow$<br>$HBuf + B^+X^-$ | Low | Low | Low |
| | Loss of $HCO_3^-$ from ECF | Loss of small-intestinal fluids: diarrhea, vomiting, suction, fistula<br>Renal loss: congenital or acquired renal tubular acidosis | $H_2CO_3 + B^+Buf^- \longrightarrow$<br>$B^+HCO_3^- + HBuf$ | | | |
| Metabolic alkalosis | Gain of strong base by ECF | Loss of $H^+Cl^-$: vomiting or suction of gastric juice<br>Loss of $H^+$ urine-F: $K^+$ depletion | $B^+OH^- + H_2CO_3 \longrightarrow$<br>$B^+HCO_3^- + HOH$<br>$B^+HCO_3^- + HBuf \longrightarrow$<br>$B^+Buf + H_2CO_3$ | High | Normal or high | High |
| | Gain of exogenous $HCO_3^-$ by ECF | Exogenous administration: ingestion of infusion of $HCO_3^-$ or bicarbonate precursors | $B^+HCO_3^- + HBuf \longrightarrow$<br>$H_2CO_3 + B^+Buf^-$ | | | |

*Reflects primary change
†Reflects compensatory change

Table 3. Etiologies and Compositional Changes in Plasma in Respiratory Acid-Base Disorders

| Disturbance | General Etiology | Clinical Examples | Buffer Reactions | Changes in Plasma | | |
|---|---|---|---|---|---|---|
| | | | | $PCO_2$* | $[HCO_3{}^-]$† | pH |
| Respiratory acidosis | Primary reduction in alveolar ventilation (primary gain of $CO_2$) | CNS: depression of respiratory center (drugs, disease)<br>Chest wall: muscle paralysis or chest wall deformity | $H_2CO_3 + B^+Buf^- \longrightarrow$ $B^+HCO_3{}^- + HBuf$ | Acute | | |
| | | | | High | Slightly high | Low |
| | | Lung: intrinsic diffuse disease (obstructive disease) | | Sustained | | |
| | | | | High | High | Low or normal |
| Respiratory alkalosis | Primary increase in alveolar ventilation (primary loss of $CO_2$) | CNS: stimulation of respiratory center (emotion, salicylate, progesterone) | $B^+HCO_3{}^- + HBuf \longrightarrow$ $H_2CO_3 + B^+Buf^-$ | Acute | | |
| | | | | Low | Slightly low | High |
| | | Reflex stimulation: hypoxemia, localized pulmonary disease<br>Other: hepatic coma | | Sustained | | |
| | | | | Low | Low | High or normal |

*Reflects primary change
†Reflects secondary change due to buffering or compensation

Blood pH is rarely, if ever, fully readjusted to normal through respiratory compensation—that is, *complete compensation* (normal blood pH) is rarely if ever achieved unless the metabolic acidosis is very mild. Respiratory compensation ameliorates the low blood pH so pH is higher than if no compensation occurred—that is, there is *partial compensation*. Definitive correction of metabolic acidosis occurs via the kidney through acidification of the urine, with a concomitant elevation of the plasma bicarbonate concentration to normal; when this is followed by respiratory readjustment of $PCO_2$, the blood acid-base status is definitely corrected to normal.

## Metabolic alkalosis

In metabolic alkalosis, the sequence is almost exactly the opposite of metabolic acidosis. The primary etiologic event in all cases is a gain of strong base or a gain of bicarbonate by the ECF. There are several clinically important etiologies for metabolic alkalosis (see Table 2). A gain of $OH^-$ by the body fluids occurs whenever there is a loss of strong acid, since the ultimate source of the $H^+$ ions being lost as strong acid is water. Thus, when hydrochloric acid is secreted by the stomach, $H^+$ ions appear in the lumen of the stomach and $OH^-$ is returned to the plasma where it is buffered by $H_2CO_3$ to form bicarbonate. Loss of $H^+Cl^-$ due to vomiting constitutes one major cause of metabolic alkalosis clinically. In pediatrics this occurs most often in infants with pyloric stenosis. Another etiology of metabolic alkalosis involving a gain of strong base is associated with potassium deficiency. In the past, there was some difference of opinion about whether potassium depletion led to metabolic alkalosis by a predominantly extrarenal mechanism or by a primary renal mechanism. In the former case, potassium was believed to leave cells in exchange for sodium and hydrogen ions, both of which were derived from the ECF. The hydrogen ions were derived from water of the ECF, and to the extent that they entered cells, *hydroxyl* ($OH^-$) ions were left behind and buffered by $CO_2$ to form bicarbonate. The other view held that the renal mechanism was primarily involved and alkalosis came about by the kidney's inappropriately secreting hydrogen ions into the urine, leaving "new" bicarbonate ions behind in the body fluids. In this view, the $H^+$ was conceived to be in competition with $K^+$ for $Na^+$ reabsorption; with $K^+$ depletion, $H^+$ secretion was formed. In either case, the result would be the same—metabolic alkalosis accompanied by potassium depletion. However, most authorities have now discarded the former view in favor of some variation of the renal theory.

The second general etiology of metabolic alkalosis involves exogenous loads of bicarbonate or bicarbonate precursors. Thus, inappropriate infusions or ingestion of large amounts of sodium bicarbonate might produce a metabolic alkalosis if the bicarbonate is not excreted by the kidney. A number of salts of organic acids—notably citrate, lactate, acetate, and gluconate—might also produce metabolic alkalosis through the provision of an exogenous bicarbonate load. This comes about because each of these organic anions can, in essence, be metabolized to $CO_2$, water, and bicarbonate:

$$C_6H_5O_7^- + 4\tfrac{1}{2}\ O_2 \longrightarrow CO_2 + 1\ H_2O + 3\ HCO_{3c}^-$$
(citrate)

$$C_3H_5O_3^- + \phantom{2}3\ O_2 \longrightarrow 2\ CO_2 + 2\ H_2O + 1\ HCO_3^-$$
(lactate)

$$C_2H_3O_2^- + \phantom{2}2\ O_2 \longrightarrow 1\ CO_2 + 1\ H_2O + 1\ HCO_3^-$$
(acetate)

$$C_6H_{11}O_8^- + \phantom{2}5\ O_2 \longrightarrow 5\ CO_2 + 5\ H_2O + HCO_3^-$$
(gluconate)

*[handwritten margin note:]* Bicarb precursors / citrate / lactate / acetate / gluconate

The ability of these substances to act as effective bicarbonate precursors relies on: (1) the ability of the circulation to deliver the substances to the site of their metabolism, and (2) the ability of the tissues to metabolize the substances to bicarbonate. The first factor is probably the more important. If bicarbonate precursors are not metabolized, they would produce very little change in acid-base status since they would behave as neutral salts. It is only when they are metabolized completely that they can provide a bicarbonate load.

In passing, note that it is very difficult to produce a sustained, significant metabolic alkalosis by the administration of even very large amounts of bicarbonate (or bicarbonate precursors) to a normal subject, since these substances must be administered with a cation, usually sodium (such as sodium bicarbonate, sodium citrate, and others). Since a normal subject has no restriction on the excretion of cations, the bicarbonate being administered will be excreted very promptly in the urine together with the cation administered with it. On the other hand, in those patients who have restrictions on cation excretion, relatively small amounts of bicarbonate or bicarbonate precursor will readily produce a significant alkalosis. The *normal* kidney can excrete enormous amounts of bicarbonate—easily several hundred milliequivalents per day.

This can be illustrated by the following example. Assume that the pH of an alkaline urine is 8.1 and the $PCO_2$ of the urine is the same as normal plasma—that is, 40 mm Hg. The $HCO_3^-$ content of such a urine can be calculated from the Henderson-Hasselbalch equation:

$$8.1 = 6.1 + \log \frac{[HCO_3^-]}{0.03 \times 40} ; [HCO_3^-] = (0.03 \times 40)$$

$$= 10^{8.1-6.1} + 1.2 \times 10^2 = 120 \text{ mEq/L}$$

Hence, 1 L of urine would contain 120 mEq/L under these assumptions. Actually, alkaline urines usually have values for $PCO_2$ considerably higher than plasma, and, accordingly, the $[HCO_3^-]$ is substantially increased under such circumstances.

In passing, it is also worth noting that a urine with a pH of 7.1, although alkaline in the usual sense, actually contains very little bicarbonate. This can be illustrated by solving the Henderson-Hasselbalch equation substituting 7.1 for pH and 40 mm Hg for $PCO_2$; the resultant $[HCO_3^-]$ is only 12 mEq/L of urine, hardly a large amount compared to the ECF bicarbonate pool.

The buffer reactions in metabolic alkalosis produce a primary increase in bicarbonate concentration (see Table 2). Respiratory compensation produces a secondary rise in $PCO_2$, but this is often poorly developed and is never complete in the sense that blood pH is restored to normal. Definitive correction of this disorder requires excretion of excess bicarbonate in an alkaline urine. Concomitant sodium, potassium, or chloride depletion limits this correction, since its achievement requires concomitant adequate intakes of these ions.

### Respiratory acidosis

Respiratory acidosis is defined as a primary disorder of the respiratory system that produces a primary increase in alveolar $PCO_2$. A number of clinically important etiologies can be involved in respiratory acidosis. These have the common denominator of effecting a primary decrease in alveolar ventilation, and this leads to a primary elevation of plasma $PCO_2$ (see Table 3). Such disorders may be classified according to the level of the respiratory system primarily affected. Thus, the disease or disorder may involve the lung itself (e.g., emphysema), the chest wall (e.g., kyphoscoliosis or myasthenia gravis), or the central regulatory mechanisms for respiration (e.g., narcotizing drugs, severe head injury).

Buffering occurs in respiratory acidosis through the nonbicarbonate system. Compositional changes in the plasma in respiratory acidosis consist of an increase in plasma $PCO_2$ and, depending on the degree of renal compensation, a slight to marked increase in plasma bicarbonate concentration. This is accompanied by a reciprocal reduction in the plasma chloride concentration that results from augmented chloride excretion as $NH_4^+$ is excreted by the kidney to acidify the urine. Blood pH may be normal in well-compensated respiratory acidosis unless the $PCO_2$ exceeds about 60 mm Hg, in which case the disorder is only partially compensated. In cases in which there is hypochloremia coupled with avid sodium conservation, the kidney may actually overcompensate the disturbance and produce an alkaline blood pH.

## Respiratory alkalosis

Respiratory alkalosis is essentially the opposite disturbance to respiratory acidosis. It occurs by virtue of some factor that causes a primary increase in alveolar ventilation; this in turn, leads to a primary fall in plasma $PCO_2$. Such a factor (see Table 3) may involve the direct stimulation of the respiratory center (e.g., salicylate intoxication or rare central nervous system lesions) or may stimulate the center by reflex via the peripheral chemoreceptors (low oxygen tension) or the stretch receptors in the lung (localized pulmonary lesions). Pregnancy is normally associated with a mild respiratory alkalosis that is thought to be due to a stimulation of the respiratory center by progesterone. Patients with advanced liver disease usually have respiratory alkalosis, especially if they are comatose; the mechanism is not clear in this instance. The commonest but most benign form of respiratory alkalosis occurs during short-lived emotional hyperventilation in those individuals who are susceptible or during an abrupt transition to high altitude in response to a low $PO_2$.

Buffering occurs in respiratory alkalosis through the nonbicarbonate systems. The compositional changes in the plasma depend on the duration of the disorder. Plasma $PCO_2$ is always low, and if an appreciable length of time has elapsed, plasma bicarbonate concentration will fall secondarily owing to renal compensation. The fall in plasma bicarbonate concentration is reciprocated by a rise in plasma chloride concentration. Blood pH is alkaline in acute respiratory alkalosis, but if renal compensation is complete, blood pH will be normal. As in the case of metabolic alkalosis, renal composition may be limited in respiratory alkalosis by concomitant deficits of sodium and potassium.

### Acid-base disturbances due to changes in ECF volume

In addition to the four disturbances discussed above, two other distinct acid-base disorders come about not by the addition or loss of acid or base but rather by an abrupt change in the volume of the ECF without a loss or gain of bicarbonate. Consider a normal ECF having normal values for bicarbonate concentration and exposed to a normal alveolar $PCO_2$. The Henderson-Hasselbalch ratio, accordingly, is 20.0/1.0 and the blood pH is therefore 7.40. If the volume of the ECF were now abruptly doubled by the infusion of any nonbicarbonate containing fluid—for example, isotonic NaCl—both the numerator and the denominator values would be diluted to the same extent so that the ratio would remain unchanged, and blood pH following the dilution would still be 7.40 (Figure 14). If such a dilution were carried out in the body, the ongoing $CO_2$ production by the tissues would raise the concentration of dissolved $CO_2$ and carbonic acid in the ECF to normal, and, accordingly, pH would fall. The fall in blood pH would in turn stimulate respiration so that the new final steady state would be a $PCO_2$ less than normal but greater than the value obtained immediately after dilution.

This disorder is known as *dilution acidosis*. Chemically it resembles partially compensated metabolic acidosis with a low plasma bicarbonate concentration and a low blood pH. This disorder would be expected to occur most frequently after the administration of large amounts of isotonic saline—a nonbicarbonate-containing fluid—to seriously dehydrated patients whose ECF volumes are markedly contracted. Expansion of such a contracted ECF volume, particularly in the presence of preexisting metabolic acidosis (say, due to diarrhea), could cause dilution acidosis and thus pose additional threat to the acid-base equilibrium of the patient.

A disturbance that is conceptually the exact opposite of dilution acidosis has also been described. It is called *contraction alkalosis* and is seen most often in edematous patients who are given one of several classes of potent diuretics—for example, ethacrynic acid—and who respond by marked urinary losses of large amounts of sodium, chloride, and water but not of bicarbonate. The stepwise sequence underlying the development of this disorder is illustrated

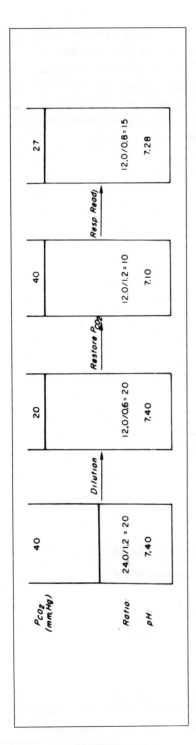

FIGURE 14. Sequence of events to explain dilution acidosis. In the first step, both numerator and denominator values are diluted to the same extent, and pH remains at 7.40. In the second step, $[CO_{2(d)} + H_2CO_3]$ is restored to normal from ongoing $CO_2$ production, and pH falls. In the third step, a secondary respiratory readjustment occurs whereby $PCO_2$ falls to a level below normal but still above that in Step 2.

in Figure 15. Extracellular fluid volume is halved, and this is followed by a second respiratory adjustment to the contraction, leading to an elevated bicarbonate concentration and blood pH.

Thus, the final result is a picture resembling partially compensated metabolic alkalosis with a high plasma bicarbonate and a high blood pH, but it has come about neither by a gain of OH⁻ nor a gain of bicarbonate but by the loss of ECF volume without a commensurate loss of bicarbonate. Theoretically this disorder should be readily corrected by the kidney through the excretion of the unwanted bicarbonate. But most patients who develop this disorder are in heart failure (this being the reason they have received the diuretics) and therefore have avid sodium conservation together with hypochloremia. Under these conditions the kidney cannot excrete the bicarbonate in an alkaline urine; thus, the disorder once produced by contraction is perpetuated, often for long periods of time.

### Mixed acid-base disturbances

Thus far, each of the so-called simple acid-base disturbances has been discussed in terms of: (1) the nature of the general causative factor, (2) the effect of that factor upon the buffer systems of the blood, (3) the nature of the secondary compensatory adjustment, and (4) the nature of the process that will correct the disturbance. In each simple acid-base disturbance, the interaction of all of these processes produces a characteristic constellation of abnormalities in blood acid-base status, the intensity of which is dependent upon the severity of the primary disorder as well as the efficacy of the compensatory and corrective mechanisms.

In conceptualizing acid-base disorders, it is useful to refer to the following qualitative expression of the Henderson-Hasselbalch equation:

$$\text{Blood pH is proportional to } \frac{\text{Metabolic component}}{\text{Respiratory component}}$$

In metabolic disorders, the responsible etiologic factor (e.g., gain of strong acid or base) affects the metabolic component *primarily*, whereas compensation affects the respiratory component as a *secondary* adjustment. In respiratory disorders, on the other hand, the opposite is true.

In contrast to these simple disorders, there is a group of disorders in which there are *two primary* independent disturbances that act on the respiratory and metabolic components simultaneously.

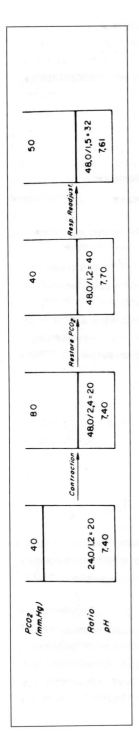

FIGURE 15. Sequence of events explaining contraction alkalosis. In the first step, both numerator and denominator values are contracted to the same extent, and pH is unaltered. In the second step, $[CO_{2(d)} + H_2CO_3]$ is restored to normal owing to "blowing off" of $CO_2$; pH rises. In the third step, a secondary respiratory adjustment occurs whereby $PCO_2$ is still elevated above normal but to a level less than that in Step 2.

47

These disorders are called *mixed* acid-base disorders. Many clinical examples of mixed disorders are conceivable, and a surprisingly large number actually occur in clinical practice. A patient manifesting diabetic ketoacidosis and concomitant pulmonary emphysema is an example of a candidate for a mixed disturbance.

Mixed disturbances pose problems with respect to terminology as well as with recognition. The terminologic issue need not be difficult, provided one abides strictly by the semantic conventions spelled out earlier (see p. 00). Hence the acid-base disorder of the patient with uncontrolled diabetes and emphysema alluded to above would likely be (mixed) metabolic acidosis and respiratory acidosis. A more confusing terminologic problem is exemplified by the mixed disturbance in the infant with severe salicylism in whom there is a direct stimulation of the respiratory center (producing respiratory alkalosis) in addition to a major abnormality in the metabolism of organic acids (producing metabolic acidosis). Here the appropriate label is mixed respiratory alkalosis and metabolic acidosis; this term seems contradictory at first glance but it is entirely consistent with the definitions of acidosis and alkalosis as abnormal physiologic processes and not as synonymous with deviations of blood pH (labelled acidemia and alkalemia, respectively). Indeed in such a mixed disturbance, blood pH may be normal, acid, or alkaline depending on the fortuitous balance between the intensity of the abnormality in the respiratory component, on the one hand, and that of the metabolic component, on the other.

The problem of diagnosis of mixed disturbances is more difficult. In essence, it involves the establishment of the presence of more than one etiologic factor as well as a physiologic interpretation of how these factors interact to produce the disorder observed in the patient. In addition, a quantitative comparison of the observed blood acid-base displacement of the patient with previously determined sets of standards drawn from patients who represent the various simple disorders (i.e., who had no independent evidence of the presence of more than one etiologic factor) is helpful, but only when it is accompanied by appropriate physiologic interpretation. For example, it is known that patients with simple metabolic acidosis show a highly predictable relationship between the degree of fall in plasma bicarbonate concentration, reflecting the primary disorder, and the degree in the fall in plasma $PCO_2$, reflecting respiratory compensation. In a given patient suspected of having a disorder known to produce metabolic acidosis, comparison of the observed blood acid-base data with this predetermined pathway tends to confirm the presence of simple metabolic acidosis if the observed data from the patient lie within this zone. But if the observed data lie outside this pathway, a mixed disturbance may be present. For example, if the observed plasma $PCO_2$ is inappropriately high in relation to the degree of fall of plasma bicarbonate, one may suspect that respiratory compensation is incomplete. This patient may therefore manifest mixed respiratory acidosis and metabolic acidosis, and a detailed search for the cause of the respiratory impairment should be undertaken. On the other hand, if the plasma $PCO_2$ is inappropriately low, some additional factor is stimulating respiration over that expected for usual compensation of metabolic acidosis. In this instance, the disorder might be mixed metabolic acidosis and respiratory alkalosis; again, this calls for a search for the cause of the disorder.

This seemingly simple method of approaching the recognition of mixed disturbances can be deceptive owing to the effects of other physiologic factors (e.g., the time needed for development of full compensation in the simple disorders) as well as the validity of the previously determined pathways used as quantitative standards. The complexities of this general subject of mixed disturbances together with the quantitative details of the expected pathways for the simple disturbances is beyond the scope of this work. The interested reader is referred to the author's other books in which this general subject is dealt with in more detailed fashion.

## WHOLE BLOOD SYSTEM OF CONCEPTUALIZING ACID-BASE PHENOMENA
### Whole blood buffers

Over the years, two different but interrelated schemes have been suggested for the conceptualization of the acid-base status of blood. Fundamentally, these two systems differ depending upon whether the base of reference is the plasma bicarbonate system alone or whether it includes all buffer systems in both phases of whole blood. The foregoing discussion of acid-base disorders has dealt exclusively with the former system. But because whole blood buffer concepts are frequently referred to in the pediatric literature, it is appropriate to summarize them here.

Since the whole blood system embraces all blood buffers, it is obviously more complex than the plasma bicarbonate system not

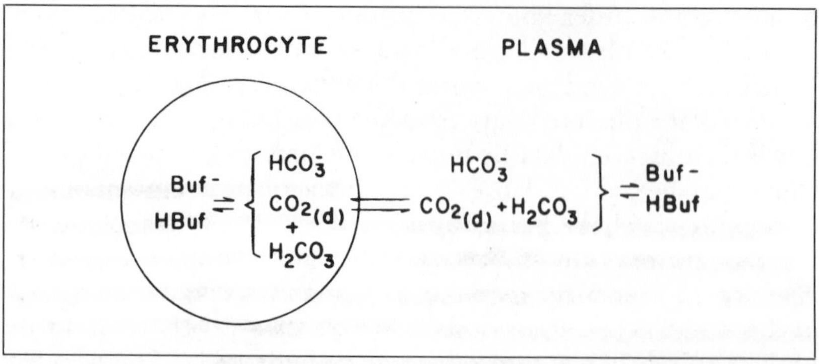

FIGURE 16. Relationships between bicarbonate and nonbicarbonate buffers in the plasma and the erythrocyte.

only because one must consider both phases of blood (i.e., plasma and erythrocyte) and their interrelationships, but also because each phase contains several buffer systems within it. In presenting this subject, it is useful to introduce the following simplifications (Figure 16): (1) to classify the buffers of each phase of blood into the bicarbonate buffer system and the nonbicarbonate buffer system, the latter consisting of inorganic phosphate and proteins in the plasma and hemoglobin, and organic and inorganic phosphate in the erythrocyte, (2) to treat all of the nonbicarbonate buffers in each phase as a single group, using the generic symbol Buf⁻ for the conjugate base forms and HBuf for the weak acid forms, and (3) to equate the nonbicarbonate buffers of blood with hemoglobin; this is justified because hemoglobin represents more than 75 percent of all the nonbicarbonate buffers of blood. It also means that for all practical purposes, Buf⁻ and HBuf of blood are restricted to the erythrocyte. This is in contrast to the bicarbonate buffer system, which is present in both phases owing to the fact that both bicarbonate and $PCO_2$ freely and rapidly pass the erythrocyte membrane.

It is this ability of both members of the bicarbonate buffer system to permeate freely that allows the plasma buffers to interact with the erythrocyte buffers. To put it another way, although the principal nonbicarbonate buffer is restricted to the erythrocyte, any factor that directly affects the plasma bicarbonate system will be reflected virtually instantaneously by the erythrocyte bicarbonate and nonbicarbonate buffer systems and vice versa. Thus, any consideration of whole blood buffering must take account of the quantitative importance of the nonbicarbonate buffers (see the buffer equations shown in Table 3).

## Blood buffer base and base excess

To further pursue the description of the whole blood buffers, it is necessary to introduce two additional concepts. The first is the concept of *whole blood buffer base* (BB), defined as the sum of the concentrations (in mEq/L) of all conjugate bases in one liter of whole blood—that is, the sum of bicarbonate and nonbicarbonate buffers in the plasma plus those in the erythrocyte:

$$BB = \underbrace{[HCO_3^-] + [Buf^-]}_{Plasma} + \underbrace{[HCO_3^-] + [Buf^-]}_{Erythrocyte}$$

Since most of the $Buf^-$ is hemoglobin, it is obvious that the value for *normal buffer base* (NBB) depends on the hemoglobin concentration. In normal blood with a hemoglobin concentration of 15 g/100 ml and a normal acid-base status (i.e., normal blood pH, normal plasma $PCO_2$, and normal plasma bicarbonate concentration), NBB is 48 mEq/L. In an anemic blood, let us say one with a hemoglobin of 10 g/100 ml, the NBB drops to 44 mEq/L. At first glance, this relatively slight fall in NBB (about 10%) seems anomalous compared with the substantial fall (33%) in hemoglobin concentration. The explanation, of course, is that as the hematocrit falls, the fraction of plasma per liter of whole blood rises; hence, the contribution of plasma bicarbonate to the total blood buffer base rises, thereby partially offsetting the effects of the reduction of $Buf^-$ to the total blood buffer base.

It follows from these considerations that the NBB for any given blood sample can be specified only in terms of its particular hemoglobin concentration. Because of this, there can be no single value for NBB applicable to all blood samples as there is, for example, for plasma sodium concentration. Rather, to be able to specify a given normal value requires a sliding scale of normal values that depend on the range of different hemoglobin values. To get around the problem this causes, a second concept was introduced that made unnecessary the use of hemoglobin concentration in determining whether a given value for blood buffer base was normal or not. This was the concept originally dubbed $\Delta BB$ and, more recently, *blood base excess* or BE. Quite simply, these two terms were defined as follows:

$$\Delta BB = BE = \text{Observed BB} - \text{normal BB}$$

This expression conveys the magnitude of the observed change in BB of a particular blood sample from the normal value for that particular blood specimen as would be appropriate for its specific hemoglobin concentration. In normal blood the observed BB equals the NBB, and $\Delta$BB and BE, therefore, are 0 mEq/L.

But suppose a patient's blood sample having a hemoglobin of 15 g/100ml had a measured BB of 52 mEq/L. Since it is known that the NBB for such a blood is 48 mEq/L:

$$\Delta BB = BE = 52 \text{ mEq/L} - 48 \text{ mEq/L} = + 4 \text{ mEq/L}$$

Suppose another patient with a hemoglobin concentration of 20 g/100 ml has an observed BB of 48 mEq/L. This is a normal value for blood with a hemoglobin of 25 g/100ml but an abnormal value for blood of 20 g/100ml in which the NBB is 44 mEq/L. In this case,

$$\Delta BB = BE = 48 \text{ mEq/L} - 44 \text{ mEq/L} = + 4 \text{ mEq/L}$$

In both of the examples, the BE of + 4 mEq/L is the amount of excess base present in each liter of blood. In other words, the blood has a *base excess* of 4 mEq/L. This is the only information conveyed by this expression. It does *not* tell us whether the excess base has accumulated owing to a direct gain of strong base or owing to a loss of acid. Nor does it tell us the physiologic mechanisms by which such an abnormality has occurred or how many liters of the patient's blood share this measured abnormality. Finally, it does not tell us whether the patient has a simple or a mixed metabolic alkalosis, a simple or mixed compensated respiratory acidosis, or a contracting alkalosis, all of which are characterized by either a primary or a compensatory increase in the base content of the blood.

If it does not tell us any of these things, what, then does it tell us? It tells us that a BE of + 4 mEq/L is an accurate estimation of the total distortion from normal in all buffers in 1 L of whole blood. This is in contrast to the less complete information given by analysis of the plasma from a whole blood sample, which shows an increase of 4 mEq/L above normal in the plasma bicarbonate concentration. In this latter case we know only the degree of distortion in one buffer system; hence, our information about the other blood buffers is less complete. But the key question— how valuable any additional information obtained by the whole blood measurements is for practical purposes—will be deferred until later.

The measured buffer base can, of course, be less than the normal buffer base in a given blood sample. Consider the following example of a blood having a hemoglobin of 15 g/100ml and a measured BB of 40 mEq/L:

$$\Delta BB = BE = 48 \text{ mEq/L} - 44 \text{ mEq/L} = + 4 \text{ mEq/L}$$

In this blood, there has been a fall in buffer base of 8 mEq/L or, to put the matter differently, the base excess is $-8$ mEq/L. The awkwardness of using a negative value for base excess has caused some clinicians to object to the use of the whole blood buffer system, but this objection can be readily overcome by using the term *base deficit*, defined as follows:

Base excess = $-$ Base deficit

Hence, if one objects to having a negative value for an excess, he can substitute a positive value for a deficit. The root of this problem is that in ordinary English usage we are much more accustomed to speaking of positive deficits than negative excesses.

### Practical usefulness of whole blood buffer system

The substantive question concerning a choice between the traditional plasma bicarbonate system and the whole blood buffer system is which system gives the most useful physiologic information for diagnosis and treatment. The answer requires an appreciation of the history of research in blood buffers. Initially, it was believed that the quantitative behavior of blood in response to addition or loss of $CO_2$ in vitro was identical to that in vivo. The relevant buffer reactions are as follows:

$$CO_2 + H_2O \longrightarrow H_2CO_3 + Buf^- \longrightarrow HBuf + HCO_3^-$$

When this reaction is studied in the left-to-right direction in vitro by the addition of $CO_2$ or in the opposite direction by the loss of $CO_2$, it was found that there was a strict reciprocal change in the amount of $Buf^-$ consumed as a reactant and the amount of $HCO_3^-$ generated as a product. Recalling that BB is defined as the sum of $Buf^- + HCO_3^-$, it follows that BB did not change after the addition or loss of $CO_2$, although, of course, the relative contributions of the two components comprising the BB did change.

If, as had been assumed for a number of years, blood in vivo behaved in exactly the same quantitative way as blood in vitro, a number of conceptual and semantic simplifications would have been possible. Had this been so, the whole blood buffer system

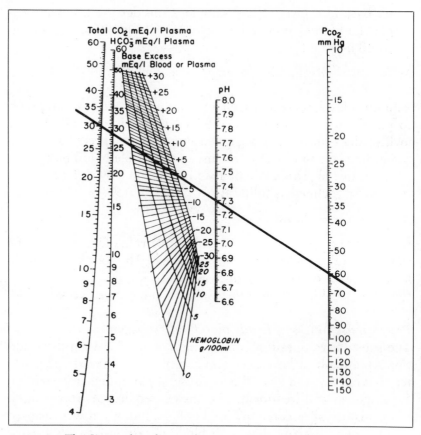

FIGURE 17. The Siggaard-Andersen alignment nomogram that quantitatively relates plasma and whole blood acid-base parameters. (The nomogram is copy-
righted by Radiometer, Copenhagen.)

would have unquestionably been a superior, albeit a more compli-
cated, base of reference since the underlying physiologic (indirectly) therapeutic principles would have been much simpler.

But careful studies of animals as well as normal human subjects
showed unequivocally that the in vitro behavior of blood differed
considerably from the in vivo behavior; thus, the potentially simplifying factors alluded to earlier were shown to be invalid.
Whereas no claim for superiority of the whole blood system can
now be sustained, one must hasten to add that no valid claim can
be sustained that this system is inferior to the plasma bicarbonate
system. In fact, both require considerable physiologic interpretation for their intelligent use in both diagnosis and treatment.

Finally, it should be recognized that the two systems are really two sides of the same coin. This is because the quantitative physiologic relationships between the plasma bicarbonate system and all the other blood buffers are so well worked out that, in effect, if one has data expressed in terms of one system, it can be neatly and accurately translated into the terms of the other system. Thus, if blood pH, plasma $PCO_2$, and hemoglobin concentration are known, the values for plasma bicarbonate, whole blood buffer base, and base excess are fixed and readily derivable. The commonest method of expressing these interrelationships is the alignment nomogram depicted in Figure 17.

# 3. Disorders of Potassium Metabolism

## NORMAL POTASSIUM BALANCE

Potassium is a major cation in the ICF, having a concentration 40 or more times that of the ECF. This much higher concentration of potassium in the cells, plus the larger volume of the ICF, means that over 98 percent of all body potassium is in the ICF. The potassium of the ICF is in dynamic equilibrium with that of the ECF by virtue of cellular membrane-active transport processes, and the ECF, in turn, is the compartment that communicates with the gastrointestinal tract and the kidneys and, hence, with the environment.

The normal adult ingests about 1 to 2 mEq of potassium per kilogram of body weight per day, and the infant may ingest several times that amount. In healthy persons, about 90 percent of the ingested potassium is absorbed from the gastrointestinal tract directly into the ECF; the remaining 10 percent appears in the stool. The constancy of the plasma potassium concentration at its normal, relatively low level in spite of the large daily intake of potassium attests to the ability of the normal regulatory and renal mechanisms to excrete potassium in the urine, thereby maintaining a normal zero balance for this ion. Dietary loads of potassium considerably larger than the usual intake may likewise be tolerated without hyperkalemia—another manifestation of the ability of the normal kidney to excrete large excesses of this ion.

Conversely, when dietary intake of potassium is markedly restricted, urinary excretion of potassium is reduced, and often after a period of several days, the renal conservation of potassium becomes quite efficient, at least in normal subjects. In general, however, the kidney seems less able to conserve potassium than sodium under severe dietary restriction. This is particularly true in disease when a whole host of factors, such as coexisting acid-base disorders, sodium excess, diuretics, intrinsic renal disease, and other factors, may limit efficient renal conservation of potassium.

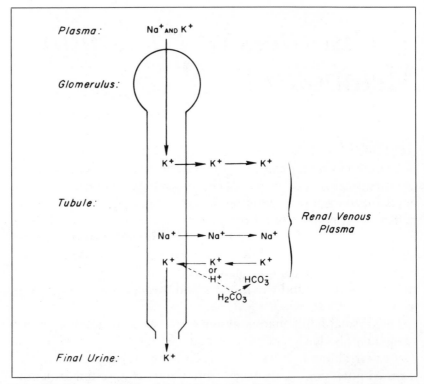

FIGURE 18. The overall role of the kidney in handling of potassium. $K^+$ filtered at the glomerulus is believed to be completely reabsorbed by the proximal tubule. In the distal tubule, $Na^+$ is reabsorbed in exchange for either $K^+$ or $H^+$, which are believed to be in competition with each other.

### Renal handling of potassium

The kidney is the major regulatory mechanism for the maintenance of potassium balance. Normally, potassium is filtered at the glomerulus, reabsorbed by the proximal tubule, and then secreted into the tubular urine by the distal nephron. Thus, the potassium ions that appear in the final urine are largely, if not entirely, those secreted by the tubules and not those filtered at the glomerulus. The secretory mechanism for potassium (Figure 18) is believed to be intimately related to the acidification mechanism of the kidney. In essence, the reabsorption of sodium ions from the tubular urine into the tubular cell and, thence, into the peritubular plasma occurs in exchange for either hydrogen ions or potassium ions secreted by the tubular cell. Hydrogen ions and potassium ions in an overall sense are in competition with each other for sodium reabsorption. Thus, when the urine is to be acidified, hydrogen ion is secreted preferentially to potassium; when bicarbonate is to be excreted (alkalinization of the urine), potassium ion secretion predominates over hydrogen, and the urine contains appreciable amounts of potassium and bicarbonate.

There are a number of factors that can affect the amount of potassium secreted in exchange for sodium that is reabsorbed. A larger-than-normal sodium load presented to the distal nephron will force the exchange mechanism, and potassium will appear in the urine in larger-than-usual quantities. It is likely that salt-retaining steroids act on the mechanism to force sodium reabsorption in exchange for potassium and, hence, to produce a decrease in sodium excretion and an increase in potassium excretion. Conversely, the lack of salt-retaining hormones limits sodium reabsorption and potassium secretion, leading to potassium retention and sodium loss such as occurs in Addison's disease. Loading the mechanisms with exogenous potassium seems to force the secretion of potassium at the expense of hydrogen ions and may, in fact, lead to a modest acidosis because of the failure of the kidney to acidify the urine. Potassium depletion, on the other hand, limits the ability of the tubular epithelium to secrete potassium; therefore, the competition with hydrogen ion is affected in favor of the latter so that the urine is acidified inappropriately, and a systemic alkalosis may result.

*Factors affecting plasma potassium concentration*
A number of factors can affect the plasma potassium concentration, the two most important being the total body potassium stores and the acid-base status of the blood. These effects are schematically represented in Figure 19. If blood pH is normal, one can expect that a fall in *total body potassium* (TBK) will be accompanied by a fall in plasma potassium concentration. The relationship is probably not strictly accurate quantitatively, but the underlying concept is valid in a qualitative sense in that the lower the TBK, the lower the plasma potassium. Alkalosis, either metabolic or respiratory, causes the plasma potassium to fall even in the absence of a deficit of TBK. But if alkalosis and body potassium depletion coexist, plasma potassium will be lower than in an equivalent degree of TBK depletion in the absence of alkalosis. Acidosis, on the other hand, tends to produce a higher than normal plasma potassium value for any value of TBK. Thus, potassium depletion may

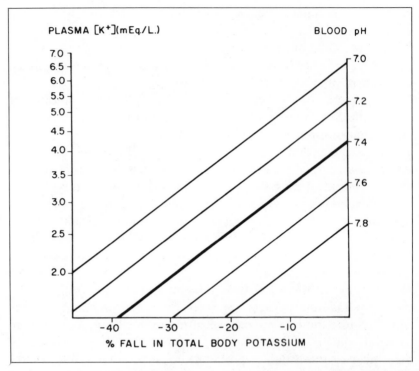

FIGURE 19. Factors affecting plasma potassium concentration. Although plasma potassium concentration falls as total body potassium falls, the level of plasma (potassium) at any given value for total body potassium will be higher than normal if blood pH is acid and lower than normal if blood pH is alkaline.

occur with a normal, or even elevated, plasma potassium if the subject is sufficiently acidotic.

## POTASSIUM DEPLETION AND EXCESS
### Potassium depletion and hypokalemia
*Potassium depletion* is defined as a loss of TBK and occurs whenever the intake of potassium is less than the output—that is, whenever there is a sustained negative balance for potassium. Most often in disease, this comes about through a combination of a low intake plus abnormal losses of potassium, occurring either through the urine (due to inefficient renal conservation secondary to any of a number of factors) or through the loss of potassium via the gastrointestinal secretions, all of which contain potassium in concentrations of 10 to 30 mEq/L. Under these conditions, potassium leaves the ICF, enters the ECF, and is lost to the environment. Potassium concentration in the ICF, therefore, falls. In order to

maintain electroneutrality in the cell, it is apparent that an intracellular anion must be lost from the cell, or the potassium loss must be matched by an equivalent transfer of an extracellular cation, such as sodium.

The first possibility—loss of intracellular anion—is unlikely since the intracellular anions are largely proteinates and organic phosphates (see Figure 3), large molecules that cannot freely pass the cell membrane. Rather, the evidence would seem to indicate that the second possibility—a gain of extracellular cation equivalent to the loss of intracellular potassium—is more likely. The main cation gained by the cells is undoubtedly sodium, and it is likely that most if not all of the intracellular cation is made up by such sodium movements. Some evidence indicates that intracellular hydrogen ion might also participate, but current evidence casts increasing doubt on this previously held hypothesis. If extracellular hydrogen ion does move into cells, it leaves a hydroxyl ion behind; this is one explanation for the occurrence of the metabolic alkalosis so often accompanying potassium deficiency. Even granting the possible existence of this mechanism, much more sodium seems to move from ECF to ICF than does hydrogen ion, and, thus, sodium is the most important ion in maintaining the electroneutrality of cells that have lost potassium.

It is important to differentiate between body potassium depletion and hypokalemia. *Body potassium depletion* is defined as a reduction in body potassium from normal—that is, a fall in intracellular potassium. It may or may not be accompanied by *hypokalemia*, which is defined as a fall in plasma potassium concentration (see Figure 19). Thus, hypokalemia can exist without significant body potassium depletion (e.g., in acute alkalosis); on the other hand, body potassium depletion can be associated with normokalemia or even hyperkalemia (e.g., in acidosis).

### Potassium excess and hyperkalemia

Whereas many disorders may lead to a deficit of body potassium with a fall of body potassium stores, there is no known disorder in which a significant sustained increase in intracellular potassium above the normal value can occur. This is to say, body potassium excess with storage of the excess potassium in cells does not occur. It is thus important to differentiate between an excess of body potassium and hyperkalemia. *Hyperkalemia* refers strictly to a higher-than-normal concentration of potassium in the plasma

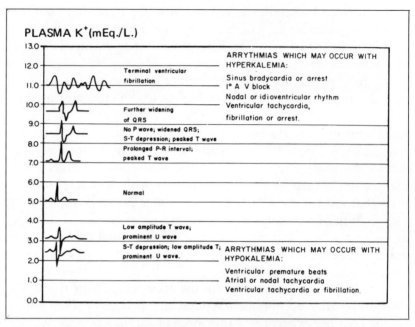

**PLASMA K⁺(mEq./L.)**

FIGURE 20. Approximate relationships between plasma potassium concentration and electrocardiographic abnormalities.

and, hence, in the ECF. Thus, if intracellular potassium stores are normal (contain 98% of the TBK), increasing the *extracellular* potassium content from the normal of 2 percent of the total body potassium to 4 percent will produce nearly fatal hyperkalemia but no significant increase in TBK. It is clear from these considerations that if body potassium stores are already normal, only a slight positive balance of potassium is needed to produce marked hyperkalemia. But, as pointed out earlier, the normal individual has an impressive ability to excrete large loads of potassium; the presence of a slight, sustained positive balance when TBK is normal implies a defect in this mechanism. If, on the other hand, body potassium stores are depleted, a large load of potassium will readily lead to an appreciable positive balance of potassium to restore the intracellular potassium deficit. It is important to note, however, that the ECF is the vehicle by which potassium is delivered from an environmental source to the cells in the restoration of such deficits. Since the potassium concentration of the ECF is normally low, to avoid serious degrees of transient hyperkalemia, safe restoration of a low intracellular potassium level (which may be as low as 60% of the normal value) requires several days.

## Effects of potassium deficiency, hypokalemia, and hyperkalemia

Depletion of body potassium, particularly when accompanied by hypokalemia, might produce changes in a number of organ systems. Of greatest importance are the effects on the heart, the neuromuscular system, and the kidney. Electrocardiographic abnormalities, shown in Figure 20, tend to accompany hypokalemia and potassium depletion, with abnormalities becoming more severe as the degree of hypokalemia and potassium depletion increases. Weakness of skeletal muscle also might occur, but it is often equivocal; frank paralysis is rare. This effect of potassium depletion on skeletal muscle might also be accompanied by a comparable effect on smooth muscle, particularly in the intestinal tract, where it might take the form of a decrease in peristalsis or paralytic ileus. A third effect of potassium depletion involves the kidney, specifically the urinary concentrating mechanism—*potassium deficiency nephropathy*. This complication tends to occur with prolonged potassium depletion and consists of the diminution or loss of the ability to produce an osmotically concentrated urine. In severe cases, overt polyuria, obligatory hyposthenuria, and secondary polydipsia may be seen. Frank morphologic changes occur in renal tubular epithelium, and the deranged kidney may be more susceptible than the normal to pyelonephritis. Repletion of body potassium stores tends to restore the concentrating defect, although there is probably some residual anatomical and, perhaps, functional change that persists.

There are no specific symptoms accompanying hyperkalemia. Changes occur in the electrocardiogram (see Figure 20). Severe degrees of hyperkalemia pose a serious threat to normal cardiac conduction, and fetal cardiac arrhythmias may occur at very high levels of plasma potassium concentration.

## Treatment of hyperkalemia

The treatment of hyperkalemia is a medical emergency because cardiac conduction may be seriously or even fatally impaired. Although the details of treatment of hyperkalemia are beyond the scope of this work, the general kinds of measures taken deserve brief comment. It is useful to list these in order of their time course of action beginning with those that are most rapid in action as follows: (1) infusion of a calcium-containing solution, (2) infusion of glucose and insulin, (3) trapping of the potassium normally present in the gastrointestinal secretions by the use of an ion exchange resin like Kayexalate, (4) use of peritoneal dialysis, and (5) use of hemodialysis. In general, the intensity of the particular hyperkalemic setting will dictate the time course and, hence, the measures that should be taken to treat the disorder.

# II. Therapy

# 4. Fluid Therapy

In approaching a patient manifesting a disorder of hydration, it is useful to separate the water and electrolyte requirements of the patient into two general phases or categories—*maintenance* requirements and *deficit* requirements. Each of these phases of fluid therapy has its own base of reference by which the requirements can be computed. Maintenance therapy consists essentially of providing water and electrolyte in amounts equal to the losses being sustained. It is also useful to differentiate between normal and abnormal losses. Thus, *normal maintenance requirements* consist of the amounts of water and electrolyte lost through the usual routes—insensible water loss, sweat, urine, and stool. In addition, any ongoing abnormal losses—that is, in abnormal amounts or through abnormal routes—should be replaced as they occur; these might be thought of as *abnormal maintenance requirements*, which, when added to the normal, give the *total maintenance requirements*.

In terms of the balance principle discussed earlier, the function of maintenance therapy is to maintain low body stores and zero balance for water, sodium, potassium, chloride, and other requirements (Figure 21). These attributes of maintenance therapy can be summarized as follows:

Normal maintenance + Abnormal maintenance = Total maintenance
= Zero balance = No change in body stores

The other phase of fluid therapy, *replacement therapy*, is the restoration of any previously incurred deficits of body stores of water, sodium, potassium, chloride, and other requirements. This process takes several days, and the patient continues to expend water and electrolyte normally through the skin, lungs, and kidneys so that normal maintenance requirements must also be provided during this period. In addition, abnormal losses may continue, and these must be replaced (as abnormal maintenance requirements). If neither of these two types of maintenance is pro-

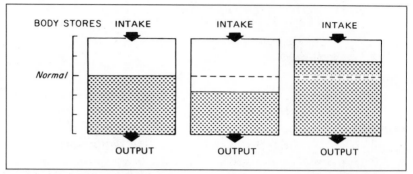

FIGURE 21. In all three diagrams, intake equals output as indicated by the wide arrows, and body stores remain constant at the existing level whether normal (*left*), low (*center*), or high (*right*).

vided, replacement therapy alone in a subject manifesting a deficit will not renew body stores; ongoing normal and abnormal losses will constitute a continuing drain on them.

Not all patients require replacement therapy, but all require maintenance therapy either orally or parenterally. For example, a well-hydrated patient hospitalized for elective surgery has no preexisting deficits, and, barring complications, should experience no abnormal maintenance requirements. The problem of fluid therapy in this case consists of the relatively simple task of providing reasonable allowances of water, sodium, potassium, chloride, and other requirements parenterally to cover the usual ongoing normal losses—in short, *normal* maintenance therapy—until an adequate oral intake can be resumed.

Maintenance and replacement therapies have separate bases of reference for computation. This is an additional reason for making the distinction between them. Specific approaches for computation of normal and abnormal maintenance requirements as well as deficit requirements will be presented in subsequent sections.

## MAINTENANCE REQUIREMENTS
### Normal maintenance requirements and their computation

The aim of maintenance fluid therapy is to provide reasonable quantities of water and electrolyte to keep the patient in zero balance. Many rules of thumb have been suggested to calculate such requirements. In general, these rules apply only to patients in specific narrow age or weight ranges and cannot be applied uniformly to all pediatric patients, who may be small premature infants or strapping adolescents. It is primarily for this reason that pediatricians have sought a more fundamental basis for determining maintenance requirements. A system based on physiologic first principles is the one adopted here. Its great advantage is that it is physiologically valid for the entire range of patient size and age and is therefore as applicable to adult medicine as to pediatric medicine.

### Normal maintenance water requirements

Fundamentally, water and electrolyte requirements for normal maintenance depend not on body size but on the rate of metabolism. That is to say, the maintenance or "wear and tear" needs are more closely related to the rate at which the metabolic engine turns over than to the weight of the engine itself.

There are fundamental physiologic reasons why metabolic rate is the primary determinant of maintenance water requirements. For example, it is not surprising that metabolic rate bears a close relationship to the insensible water loss (IWL), since the metabolic rate determines the heat production of the body and the IWL is an important means of ridding the body of heat. Thus, approximately 45 ml of water is lost through the skin and lungs as IWL for each 200 Calories (Cal) expended. The reader is reminded that 1 *Calorie* (so-called large calorie or kilocalorie) is equivalent to 1000 small calories. Of this 45 ml, about one third is lost through the lungs as pulmonary water loss, while the remaining two thirds is lost through the skin.

The other main route of maintenance water loss is the urine. Since urinary volume can vary within wide limits, no single value can be selected as the ideal normal. But the general case can be made that urinary volume is also related to metabolic rate in an approximate way, since metabolism determines the amount of endogenously generated solute presented to the kidney for excretion. However, urinary volume also varies with the intake of exogenous solutes (e.g., largely electrolytes) as well as with the need of the organism to conserve or to excrete water. Figure 22 shows a plot of the urinary volume over the possible range of urine concentration the human kidney can achieve. If the renal solute load, which consists of both endogenous and exogenous solutes, is high (e.g., 40 mOsm/100 Cal expended), urinary volume will be greater at any given urinary osmolarity than if the solute excretion is low. In formulating maintenance requirements for urinary volume, the aim is to select a reasonable value that will cover most situations without unduly taxing either the diluting or the concentrating

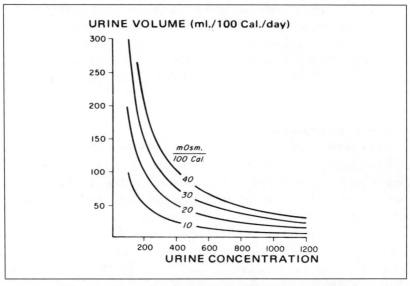

FIGURE 22. Urinary volume as a function of urinary concentration for various solute loads, varying from high (40 mOsm/100 Cal) to low (10 mOsm/100 Cal). If urine volume were 55 ml/100 Cal, the high solute load could be excreted at a urinary concentration of about 800 mOsm/L; a low solute load would be excreted at a urine concentration of about 200 mOsm/L. Neither would tax the minimum (about 50 mOsm/L) or maximum (about 1400 mOsm/L) concentrating power of the normal kidney.

ability of the kidney and be capable of handling extremes of solute excretion varying from a high of 40 mOsm/100 Cal to a low of 10 mOsm/100 Cal. A value of 55 ml/100 Cal expended seems a reasonable figure to meet all the requirements.

For most normal maintenance requirements, losses of water via the sweat or in formed stools can be ignored. Thus, hospitalized patients in air-conditioned rooms do not ordinarily sweat, but if ambient temperature controls are not available, some allowance should be made for sweat losses. Ordinarily, moderate sweating is associated with losses of water from 10 to 25 ml/100 Cal expended; with heavy thermal sweating, these losses may reach values of 50 ml or more per 100 Cal. Stool losses of water can usually be ignored in patients receiving parenteral fluid maintenance therapy, since they have little or no stool volume. If diarrhea is present, it should be treated as an abnormal maintenance requirement and computed separately, as explained next.

The hidden sources of water intake, as explained, can likewise be ignored in most instances. The water of oxidation is clearly a

TABLE 4. Components of Normal Maintenance Water
Requirements (ml/100 Cal)

| | |
|---|---:|
| Output | |
| Insensible water loss | 45 |
| Sweat | 0–25 |
| Urine | 50–75 |
| Stool water | 5–10 |
| Hidden intake | |
| Water of oxidation | 12 |
| Usual requirement in absence of sweating | 100 |

function of metabolic rate and averages about 12 ml/100 Cal expended, whereas preformed water intake is present only when there is extensive tissue catabolism. Such sources of water need to be considered and subtracted from the intake only when one is dealing with severe oliguric renal failure.

Thus, under normal conditions, one can derive an average normal maintenance water requirement by summing the requirements for insensible water loss and urine (Table 4)—that is, approximately 100 ml/100 Cal expended. In the presence of sweating, an additional 10 to 25 ml/100 Cal should be added.

*Normal maintenance electrolyte requirements*
Since the normal kidney has a wide range of latitude for electrolyte excretion, no single figure for maintenance requirements of sodium, potassium, or chloride can be cited. Rather, as in the case of water, it is the aim of normal maintenance therapy to provide reasonable quantities of these substances—amounts that will not tax the ability of the kidney to excrete a large excess or force maximal conservation to preserve diminished body stores. One method of deriving such requirements is to examine the usual oral electrolyte intake of the healthy infant and to express it in terms of the caloric intake, which in turn closely approximates the caloric expenditure of the infant. Hence, one may compare the electrolyte intake of human milk with that of a cow's milk formula, both expressed per 100 Cal fed. Human milk provides relatively low intakes of electrolytes, averaging about 1 to 1.5 mEq/100 Cal for sodium and potassium; a cow's milklike formula provides two to three times more. Since both types of feedings are known to be adequate for normal infants, a reasonable figure can be arrived at simply by splitting the difference and providing approximately 2.5 mEq each of sodium and potassium per 100 Cal expended. These

electrolytes can be provided exclusively as the chloride salts; that is, sodium chloride and potassium chloride—giving a slight "excess" for chloride. Such a small amount of excess chloride is not likely to be important, since the total chloride intake is not large in the maintenance fluids.* This problem of excess chloride is more important in replacement fluids, as will be discussed in the following paragraphs.

### Normal maintenance caloric requirements

Ideally, one would like to provide 100 Cal of foodstuffs for every 100 Cal expended by the patient. Using the parenteral route exclusively, this can be accomplished by using mixtures of amino acids, fat, and carbohydrate together with all other nutrients delivered via the central venous route (see Chapter 5, Parenteral Nutrition). In patients with short-term illness and no preexisting malnutrition, it is not necessary to attempt to provide full caloric replacement, since adequate depot fat stores are usually present to make up the difference between a short-term suboptimal exogenous caloric intake and the ongoing caloric expenditure. Rather, a more modest goal is to provide enough glucose to prevent ketosis and to minimize endogenous protein breakdown. This amount of glucose is approximately 20 percent of the total caloric expenditure. In other words, 20 Cal from glucose should be provided for each 100 Cal expended by the patient. Since 1 g of glucose supplies about 4 Cal, this requirement corresponds to 5 g of glucose per 100 Cal expended by the patient.

### Summary of normal maintenance requirements

Based on the foregoing, normal maintenance requirements can be defined on the basis of caloric expenditure of the patient as follows:

Water      = 100 to 125 ml/100 Cal expended
Sodium     = 2.5 mEq/100 Cal expended
Potassium  = 2.5 mEq/200 Cal expended
Glucose    = 5 g/100 Cal expended

It is obvious that these recommendations are reasonable averages drawn from a physiologic analysis. They are *not* to be construed as unalterably precise; rather, since the organism has such great

---

*A recent unfortunate experience in which batches of soy-based formula were inadvertently manufactured almost totally devoid of chloride with a resultant metabolic alkalosis constitutes a vivid example of the essentiality of this ion for normal physiology.

TABLE 5. Solution for Normal Maintenance Requirements

| | H$_2$O (ml) | Na$^+$ (mEq) | K$^+$ (mEq) | Cl$^-$ (mEq) | Dextrose (gm) |
|---|---|---|---|---|---|
| Mixture for 1 Liter Dextrose 5% in saline 0.9% | 165 | 25 | 0 | 25 | 8.3 |
| Potassium chloride (20 mEq/ 10 ml)* | 12.5 | 0 | 25 | 25 | 0 |
| Dextrose 5% in water (q.s. to make 1 liter) | 822.5 | 0 | 0 | 0 | 41.1 |
| Total | 1000.0 | 25 | 25 | 50 | 49.4 |

*Should be omitted if there is a possibility of inducing hyperkalemia (see precautions in potassium administration p. 146).

tolerance, any figure for water and electrolyte maintenance within a reasonable range of those listed is likely to be satisfactory unless there are specific defects in the normal regulatory mechanisms governing water and electrolyte metabolism as discussed later (see p. 75).

In general, a fluid for normal maintenance purposes should: (1) be hypotonic with respect to electrolytes, (2) contain sodium and potassium in roughly the amounts shown here, and (3) contain 5 g/100 ml or more of glucose. Any of the commercially available solutions meeting or approximating these needs may be used. Alternatively, a solution can be tailor-made precisely to these specifications (Table 5). A discussion of commercially available as well as tailor-made solutions for use in meeting maintenance purposes is presented later.

*Estimate of caloric expenditure*

Having defined requirements for normal maintenance per 100 Cal expended, it is necessary to estimate the caloric expenditure of the patient. For example, if the caloric expenditure of a given patient were known to be 500 Cal per day, maintenance requirements would be met by 500 ml of a suitable maintenance solution. A fairly accurate prediction of caloric expenditure can be made for patients weighing more than 3 kg from the measured body weight. Figure 23 shows the relationship between the number of Cal expended per 24 hr for bed patients and the body weight of the

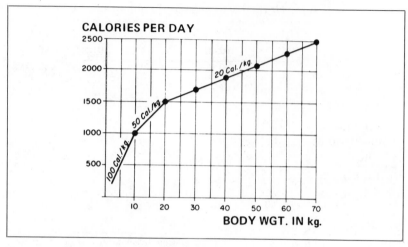

FIGURE 23. The approximate relationship between body weight and estimated caloric expenditure. The curve can be divided into three segments according to its slope: from 3 to 10 kg = 100 Cal/kg; from 10 to 20 kg = 50 Cal/kg; over 20 kg = 20 Cal/kg. These slopes can be used to formulate an estimate of caloric expenditure without use of the graph. Estimated caloric expenditure for a 25-kg patient, for example is

$$
\begin{aligned}
&\text{100 Cal/kg for each of the first 10 kilograms (10 kg} \times \text{100 Cal/kg)} = \text{1000 Cal/day}\\
&\text{50 Cal/kg for each kilogram between 10 and 20 (10 kg} \times \text{50 Cal/kg)} = \text{500 Cal/day}\\
&\text{20 Cal/kg for each kilogram over 20 (5 kg} \times \text{20 Cal/kg)} = \text{100 Cal/day}\\
&\qquad\qquad\qquad\qquad\qquad\qquad\quad \text{Total 25 kg} = \text{1600 Cal/day}
\end{aligned}
$$

patient. (The problems of the low-birth-weight infant are discussed separately; see page 80). The curve emphasizes that the younger the patient, the higher the metabolic rate per kilogram of body weight and, therefore, the higher the maintenance water and electrolyte requirements. For example, in the range of 3 to 10 kg of body weight, caloric expenditure averages about 100 Cal per kilogram, so that a child of 20 kg in bed has an estimated caloric expenditure of 1000 Cal per day and would require 1000 ml of a maintenance solution. This may be compared to the 70 kg adult bed patient whose estimated daily caloric expenditure is about 2500 Cal and who would require 2.5 liters of maintenance fluid per day. Thus, although the 70-kg adult's weight is sevenfold that of the child, the difference in maintenance requirements is less than threefold.

The values for estimated caloric expenditure calculated from the graph (Figure 23) include basal metabolic expenditure plus an average increment for activity in bed. In certain instances, this initial estimate can be refined further to take account of specific hypermetabolic or hypometabolic situations. These are summarized in Table 6. The most common cause of hypermetabolism is fever.

TABLE 6. Conditions Altering Usual Estimate of Metabolic Rate

| Condition | Type of Adjustment to be Made |
|---|---|
| *Increase in metabolic rate* | |
| Fever | Increase caloric estimate by 12% per °C rise in body temperature |
| Hypermetabolic states (hyper-thyroidism, salicylism) | Increase caloric estimate 25–75% |
| *Decrease in metabolic rate* | |
| Hypothermia | Reduce caloric estimate by 12% per °C fall in body temperature |
| Hypometabolic states | Reduce caloric estimate 10–15% |

Thus, suppose a child weighing 5 kg has fever averaging 40°C. His estimated caloric expenditure would be 500 Cal (from the graph) plus 24 percent of 500 Cal (for the 2°C of fever as shown in Table 6), giving a total of 620 Cal per day. Accordingly, maintenance requirements would be 620 ml of maintenance solution per day. Hypermetabolism from causes other than fever, as well as hypometabolic states, requires appropriate adjustment, as is shown in Table 6.

These considerations serve to emphasize the value of relating maintenance requirements to caloric expenditure because they tend to focus attention directly upon the primary factors that alter metabolic rate and, therefore, alter maintenance requirements. As such, this sytem is conceptually superior to others that are based on a sliding scale of body weight or on estimated body surface area since it will more likely lead to the identification of individual exceptions to the general rule, thereby improving and individualizing care of patients.

It should be emphasized that no one base of reference can claim greater accuracy than any other. The choice, therefore, has to be made on other grounds; metabolic rate seems to be clearly superior to all others since it is physiologically the most fundamental.

*Abnormal maintenance requirements*
There are a number of situations in which abnormal maintenance requirements must be taken into account. The general rule in such cases is to replace the abnormally lost volume with a similar volume of fluid having an electrolyte composition resembling that lost. This is most easily accomplished in the case of replacement of gastric or intestinal fluids removed by suction; the volume of fluid removed can be measured in a graduated suction bottle, and its

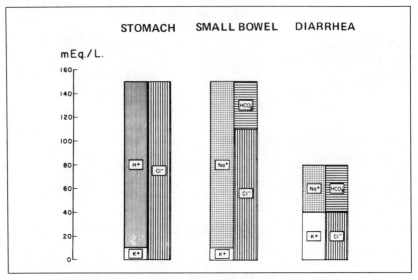

FIGURE 24. Approximate electrolyte composition of various gastrointestinal secretions.

composition can be measured directly by the laboratory or approximated from the known composition of gastric or intestinal fluids (Figure 24). Although the assumption of representative values for various constituents is usually satisfactory for small losses, direct laboratory analysis of the loss is always preferable.

The only measurements needed are those of the sodium, potassium, and chloride concentrations as well as the volume of fluid collected over a known time interval. In small-intestinal fluids, the sum of $[Na^+] + [K^+] - [Cl^-]$ will probably be a positive number and represents bicarbonate. In gastric juice, this calculation may well yield a negative number representing $[H^+]$. Once these data are in hand, a solution can be formulated to match the analytically determined values. For gastric juice, however, sodium should be substituted for the (assumed) content of $H^+$. In patients with large losses, repeated analyses may be necessary to match intake with loss.

Although the fluids of the intestinal tract are isotonic when secreted, they usually undergo dilution from swallowing hypotonic saliva, and ingestion of small amounts of water or ice chips. Thus, when they are removed and analyzed they are rarely isotonic. This is a further compelling reason for direct measurement of such losses, particularly if they are large. If assumed values are used, gastric losses should probably be replaced volume for volume by a fluid containing approximately 100 mEq/L of sodium, 15 mEq/L of potassium, and 115 mEq/L of chloride (to take account of the dilution indicated above). Small-intestinal secretions, on the other hand, should be replaced volume for volume with a fluid containing sodium, 100 mEq/L, potassium, 15 mEq/L, bicarbonate, 40 mEq/L, and chloride 75 mEq/L. Commercially available fluids for these purposes are discussed in Chapter 5 (see p. 163). Solutions tailor-made to the measured losses are obviously preferable to those available commercially.

Abnormal maintenance requirements due to ongoing diarrhea are more difficult to meet, since the volume of the stool is not readily measurable. In many instances of infantile diarrhea, however, the diarrhea promptly ceases when all oral feedings are withheld, and the problem is thereby avoided. When diarrhea does not cease, a rough approximation of stool volume can be made according to the severity of the diarrhea as shown in Table 7. The electrolyte composition of stool water in infantile diarrhea is quite variable, but it is characteristically hypotonic, with average values of about 40 mEq/L each for sodium, potassium, chloride, and bicarbonate (Figure 24). A replacement fluid containing ions in these concentrations can be readily mixed, or a commercially available solution close to this composition can be used.

The measured osmolarity of stool water is close to the isotonic value of 280 mOsm/L despite the fact that the electrolytes account for only about 160 mOsm/L (40 mOsm/L each from $Na^+$, $K^+$, $Cl^-$ and $HCO_3^-$). The unexplained osmols are probably made up of various carbohydrates and intermediates produced by bacterial metabolism. This seems to be the case when the diarrhea occurs in a child who is being fed father than fasted. But in cholera in contrast to the types of diarrhea encountered in the United States, the situation is very different, and the electrolytes account for nearly all the measured osmolarity of the stool water.

When abnormal maintenance losses are occurring via the kidney owing to some defect in regulation or to intrinsic renal disease, determining the loss accurately by measurement is preferable to estimating it. In conducting this urine collection, it is essential to have the patient on a known intake of ions and water and also to study the patient in a metabolically steady state. If these requirements are not met, the data may be uninterpretable or misleading. An example of direct assessment would be the measurement of urinary volume with known water and solute intake in a case of nephrogenic diabetes insipidus so as to provide an estimate of

TABLE 7. Conditions Affecting Abnormal Maintenance Requirements

| Factor Affected | Type of Adjustment to be Made |
| --- | --- |
| Insensible water loss requirements | |
| High environmental humidity | Reduce IWL 0–15 ml/100 Cal |
| Hyperventilation | Increase IWL 50–60 ml/100 Cal |
| Sweat requirements | |
| Mild to moderate thermal sweating in otherwise normal subject | Increase water allowance by 10–25 ml/100 Cal; increase Na$^+$ and Cl$^-$ allowance by 0.5–1.0 mEq/100 Cal |
| Mild to moderate thermal sweating in cystic fibrosis | Increase water allowance by 10–25 ml/100 Cal; increase Na$^+$ and Cl$^-$ allowance 1–2 mEq/100 Cal |
| Urine requirement | |
| Obligatory oliguria | Adjust urine water allowance to replace output |
| Obligatory polyuria | Increase urine water allowance to replace output |
| Na$^+$ or K$^+$ retaining states | Reduce or eliminate Na$^+$ or K$^+$ intake |
| Na$^+$ or K$^+$ wasting states | Increase Na$^+$ or K$^+$ intake to equal measured losses |
| Gastrointestinal losses | |
| Gastric loss | Replace volume for volume with appropriate solution |
| Small intestinal loss | Replace volume for volume with appropriate solution |
| Diarrheal loss | Replace with equal volume of appropriate solution |

the extra water needed to sustain the augmented urine volume. Similarly, if sodium-losing or potassium-losing renal disorders are present, a 24-hour measurement of sodium or potassium excretion on a known intake will provide a reasonable guideline for the amounts of these ions required to augment the intake to maintain zero balance. Obviously, the intakes of these ions should approach those the patient would be ingesting after discharge from the hospital.

Certain disorders require downward scaling of normal maintenance requirements. Thus, in edematous states, sodium is conserved, and little sodium need be provided in the intake unless there are significant extrarenal losses. In infants placed in high humidity environments, IWL through the skin and lungs may be decreased, because water cannot be evaporated into an environment already saturated with water vapor. Similarly, in patients with potassium retention, potassium should be reduced or withheld entirely from the maintenance fluids; in states of obligatory oliguria, such as those accompanying inappropriate antidiuretic hormone secretion, acute tubular necrosis, and other states, a substantial reduction in water requirements for urinary volume should be made. In general, in these cases, it is best to measure urine volume and to replace the comparable volume.

*Summary of maintenance requirements*
The foregoing discussion of maintenance requirements, both normal and abnormal, may be summarized as a series of questions that should be answered if one is to ascertain the appropriate maintenance fluid and electrolyte requirements for a particular patient:

1. Is insensible water loss allowance likely to be normal? It may be reduced with high environmental humidity (10 to 20 ml/100 Cal); it may be increased with marked hyperventilation, as in metabolic acidosis, and other states (50 to 60 ml/100 Cal).
2. Is the normal allowance for urine volume likely to be adequate? It should be reduced in states of obligatory oliguria and increased in states of obligatory polyuria. In either case, it is desirable to measure the urinary volume and to supply an equal quantity of water (plus the amount for IWL).
3. Is sweating present? If so, appropriate estimates should be made using Table 8 as a guide. If not, it can be dismissed.
4. Are abnormal gastrointestinal losses present? If gastrointestinal secretions are being lost, they should be replaced volume for volume with fluids similar in composition (Table 7). Direct analysis of the electrolyte composition of the lost fluid is preferable to the assumption of its composition.
5. Are abnormal sodium-losing and potassium-losing states present? If so, measure daily excretion of these ions on a known intake, and replace the loss by augmenting the intake appropriately.
6. Are sodium-retaining or potassium-retaining states present? If so, the sodium or potassium intake should be reduced or eliminated.
7. Is metabolic rate likely to be that expected for an uncompli-

TABLE 8. Components of Water Requirement for Preterm Infants

| Losses | ml/kg/day | |
|---|---|---|
| | VLBW (<1500 g) | LBW (>1500 g) |
| Basal insensible water loss | 30–60 | 15–35 |
| Urine | 50–100 | 50–100 |
| Stool | 5–10 | 5–20 |
| Total* | 85–170 | 70–145 |
| Phototherapy | 20 | |

*Additional increments may be needed for increases in metabolic rates secondary to cold stress, usual activity, or serious illness (e.g., sepsis, respiratory distress syndrome). Final totals may well be as follows:

| < 1000 g | > 200 ml/kg/day |
|---|---|
| 1000–1500 g | 175–200 ml/kg/day |
| 1500–2500 g | 150–200 ml/kg/day |

*Source:* Adapted from R. N. Roy and J. C. Sinclair. Hydration of the low birth weight infant. *Clin. Perinatol.* 2:393–417, 1975.

cated bed patient? If so, estimate caloric expenditure from Figure 23. If not, make appropriate adjustments using Table 6 as a guide.

## FLUID THERAPY FOR THE LOW BIRTH WEIGHT INFANT

Maintenance fluid therapy for the *low birth weight* (LBW) infant, arbitrarily defined as a birth weight of 1500 to 2500 g, and for the *very low birth weight* (VLBW) infant (birth weight less than 1500 g) deserves special consideration. These special features which are in a sense modifications of the above general physiologic approach, are mandated in these smaller infants because of a combination of physiologic regulatory handicaps along with the effects of several commonly used caretaking practices. Together, these two factors serve to alter requirements as well as to limit tolerances for water, electrolytes, and glucose, especially in the VLBW infant.

### Water requirement

Considering the water requirement first, account must be taken of the fact that metabolic rate, which is a major determinant of the IWL, is itself peculiarly sensitive to ambient temperature in the preterm infant. For this reason, it is now a nearly universal practice to servocontrol the environmental temperature to produce a thermoneutral environment for the infant, the thermoneutral environment being defined as that temperature at which oxygen consumption is minimal. It follows that any maneuver that requires the incubator to be opened will alter the thermoneutrality of the incubator and hence the metabolic rate and the IWL.

Insensible water loss is also affected by such caretaking practices as the use of radiant heaters, phototherapy, and high ambient humidity. Finally, gestational age itself seems to alter IWL; VLBW infants generally need considerably greater allotments of water for this purpose than do the heavier LBW infants. Whether this effect is related directly to metabolic rate is not clear.

With all these potential variables at work, it follows that no precise estimate can be reached for the IWL requirement of any given infant. However, assuming minimal physical activity (and activity for LBW and VLBW infants is characteristically considerably less than in term infants) and a servocontrol thermoneutral environment in a single-walled incubator having a relative humidity of approximately 50 percent, reasonable ranges of IWL can be arrived at for the VLBW and the LBW infants. These are shown in Table 8. An additional increment for phototherapy-induced skin losses is also shown. (The extra losses incident to phototherapy-induced diarrhea will be discussed later.)

The conceptual approach to defining urinary water requirements for the VLBW and the LBW infants is similar to that outlined previously for older patients—to define a volume or range of volumes that, within the definable range of solute excretion, will not unduly tax either the diluting or the concentrating mechanisms of the kidney of such premature infants. Actually, most of the evidence suggests that the renal diluting and concentrating functions are not severely limited in such infants, but the amount of solute excreted might be large, depending on the circumstances. Hence, a wider range for renal water requirement seems reasonable. See Table 8 and Author's Notes 1, page 161.

Stool water loss in sick infants who require parenteral fluid therapy is usually very small, barring some gastrointestinal problem. Infants receiving phototherapy often develop diarrhea that is attributed to a shortened transit time induced by photodecomposition products of bilirubin. The magnitude of such losses may be significant—15–20 ml/kg/day; like other abnormal losses, it should be measured, if possible, by weighing diapers and replaced volume for volume with a hypotonic electrolyte solution.

Table 8 summarizes reasonable ranges for the total water requirement and identifies the major components comprising the total. One frequent question concerns the relationships between postnatal weight loss and the need for providing some or all of the water and electrolyte requirements (see following paragraphs) during this phase. Since it is generally agreed that the weight loss experienced by all infants in the immediate postnatal period is largely water (accompanied by losses of potassium and, especially, sodium), it is unclear how much the two major compartments (ECF and ICF) share in the total.

It is noteworthy that the smaller infants lose a much larger proportion of their body weight (up to 20%) than do term infants (about 5%). Formerly, it was widely assumed that infants were born with a surfeit of water, and it followed that it was safe to withhold all fluids for the first several days. Closer study of this practice, however, showed that fasting and thirsting led to signs of dehydration often accompanied by the development of an impressive degree of hypernatremia. The early provision of calories has also been shown convincingly to be beneficial.

The problem is to define the acceptable degree of weight loss, especially in the VLBW infant whose loss is proportionately so large. It is likely to be very difficult to entirely prevent this phenomenon, but it is unsafe to neglect it. A reasonable goal would appear to be the prevention of clinical and biochemical signs of dehydration and the effects of starvation by the early provision of water, sodium, and glucose beginning 4 to 6 hours after birth, realizing that such therapy will reduce the degree of weight loss but will not abolish it. Thus, an acceptable weight loss of less than 10 percent in LBW infants and less than 15 percent in VLBW infants seems to be a reasonable practical goal.

It is interesting that if one provides total parenteral nutrition beginning on the first day of life, the postnatal weight loss in preterm infants can be almost entirely prevented. This is, of course, not necessary in the otherwise healthy LBW or VLBW infant, but it is a curious and as yet unexplained observation that must ultimately be taken into account in explaining the physiologic dynamics of postnatal weight loss in infants.

### Electrolyte requirements

The limits of sodium and potassium conservation, not clearly defined for term infants, are much less for those of lower birth weight. The available evidence, however, suggests that VLBW infants, especially, may require larger sodium intakes than would have been predicted from requirements of older infants. This may be related to those observations that tend to show that LBW infants excrete relatively large amounts of sodium even when they are hyponatremic. Whether this is a primary renal or an endocrine-mediated phenomenon is unknown. LBW infants generally will maintain normal plasma sodium concentrations on an intake of 3 mEq/kg/day. However, the VLBW infants, especially those at the very low end of the spectrum, *may* require very much larger intakes—as much as 12 to 15 mEq/kg/day in occasional instances. Under these conditions, one must be guided by frequent serial monitoring of the plasma sodium concentration in relation to the water and sodium intake as well as the hydration status in order to define the appropriate intake.

The exogenous requirement for potassium poses a different problem, judged by the infrequency of hypokalemia in the preterm infant receiving parenteral fluids (unless, of course, the parenteral regimen is nutritionally complete, and, as a result, growth is being induced—see the following paragraphs). Perhaps the reason is that very sick infants generally have a concomitant acidosis, and this drop in blood pH tends to keep the plasma potassium concentration at a normal or even an elevated level. Nevertheless, it would seem prudent to provide some potassium (1 to 2 mEq/kg/day) if there is stable renal function and plasma potassium concentration is not elevated. Serial monitoring of the clinical stability as well as of the plasma potassium concentration and blood acid-base status are the best guidelines to the amount to be given. All precautions for administering potassium must be assiduously observed in such infants.

*Glucose requirement*
The desirability of initiating early glucose feedings orally, when possible, and parenterally when not, has been adequately demonstrated. There is, however, a considerable risk to glucose loads, especially in the VLBW infants, owing to the rather severe limitation on the metabolic disposition of glucose. Studies of this phenomenon have shown that infusions of glucose delivering greater than 4 to 6 mg/kg/min readily lead to hyperglycemia. With infusion rates greater than this range, the most extreme example occurring in central venous infusion of total parenteral nutrition mixtures containing 20 percent glucose delivered at a rate of 125 ml/kg/day, the VLBW infants have often been found to have blood glucose levels that are severely elevated—in the range of 1500 to 2000 mg/100 ml in such infants, a syndrome of hyperosmolar

coma and death has been described. Even infusions of the usual volumes of 10 percent glucose and, occasionally, even 5 percent glucose may produce significant hyperglycemia in the VLBW infants. Given this lability of glucose tolerance of the VLBW infant coupled with the relatively wide range of water requirements, it is essential that the rate of glucose intake of a proposed maintenance solution be computed and expressed in mg/kg/min and checked against the safe range of 4 to 6 mg/kg/min prior to starting the infusion.

## General comments

The number of physiologic variables encountered in the preterm infant imply that extraordinarily wide ranges of water and sodium intake may be needed. Few commercially available premixed solutions are likely to be appropriate for parenteral fluid therapy of the sick LBW and VLBW infants. Rather, tailor-made solutions are needed, the compositions of which are based on the information available; subsequent modifications should be made on the basis of clinical and chemical feedback information. It is helpful to first define the requirement over a given period of time for each constituent (water, sodium, potassium, and glucose) and to summarize these in the form of a fluid prescription. Mixing of the presented fluid should then be carried out under a laminar flow hood by a trained pharmacist. Because conditions often change so rapidly in the preterm infant, it is preferable to plan fluid therapy over short time segments—for example, 6 or 8 hr—and to bracket each segment by appropriate clinical and feedback information on the basis of which the fluid prescription for the next segment of time can be generated.

Nowhere in pediatric fluid therapy is the sloppy practice of relating the fluid or intake of a patient solely as a concentration more fraught with danger than in the present setting. The amount of each constituent delivered to a patient during a stated period of time is obviously the volume of infusate over a particular time interval times the concentration of each constituent in the infusate. Thus a VLBW infant could easily be receiving a 5% glucose solution—seemingly a safe concentration—but if the volume being given were 200 ml/kg/day, which is not unreasonable, the total glucose load delivered would be 7 mg/kg/min and therefore likely to produce hyperglycemia.

Fluid therapy of the type outlined is appropriate in the LBW or the VLBW infant for a period of only a few days. If a satisfactory enteral intake cannot be established during this period, it is advisable to change to a regimen of total parenteral nutrition that will provide amino acids, minerals, vitamins, trace minerals, and essential fatty acids as well as water, calories, and electrolytes (see Chapter 5, Parenteral Nutrition). Certainly, the TPN regimen should be instituted immediately in any infant in whom an initial decision can be made that the parenteral route will be needed for 3 or more days.

## ANALYSIS OF DEFICITS
### Origin of deficits

Deficits of body water, sodium, and potassium can occur in a wide variety of clinical disorders, all of which are characterized by a negative balance of these substances over some preexisting time interval. In the simplest (but rarest) case, these negative balances occur owing to lack of any oral intake in the face of ongoing normal losses through the skin, lungs, and kidneys. In more complex cases, these normal losses are augmented by some type of abnormal (usually gastrointestinal) loss and are only partially replaced by a concomitant oral intake. Whatever the precise contributions of the various types of losses in the output and the magnitude of any concomitant intake, the syndromes of dehydration with sodium and potassium depletion signify that at some previous time the total output has always exceeded the total intake.

A completely analogous analysis applies to the pathogenesis of malnutrition in which there has been a sustained negative balance of calories or protein; this is often due to an inadequate intake, but is aggravated to a considerable degree by ongoing abnormal losses as well. A sustained negative energy balance leads to a loss of body fat, whereas a similar negative balance of nitrogen leads to a depletion of lean body tissue. However, deficits of water and electrolyte often may occur in a matter of a few days; significant deficits of fat or lean body mass generally take weeks or longer to become clinically obvious. In chronic illnesses, nutritional deficits often coexist with concomitant deficits of fluid and electrolyte, and, therefore, the nutritional as well as the hydration problems must be given consideration.

Viewed in these terms, the consequences of the depletion of water, sodium, and potassium can be examined in fundamental physiologic terms and in a form applicable, with minor modification, to any clinical disorder that may have caused the deficits. In other words, if one views the consequences of these negative bal-

TABLE 9. Probable Values of Water and Electrolyte Deficits for Moderate to Severe Dehydration in Infants

| Type of Dehydration | Range of Plasma [Na$^+$] (mEq/L) | Water (ml/kg) | Na$^+$ (mEq/kg) | K$^+$ (mEq/kg) | Cl$^-$ + HCO$_3$$^-$ (mEq/kg) |
|---|---|---|---|---|---|
| Isotonic | 130–150 | 100–150 | 7–11 | 7–11 | 14–22 |
| Hypertonic | >150 | 120–170 | 2–5 | 2–5 | 4–10 |
| Hypotonic | <130 | 40–80 | 10–14 | 10–14 | 20–28 |

ances from a fundamental physiologic viewpoint, the therapy for the successful replacement of water, sodium, and potassium depletion becomes essentially independent of the specific disease process. This is an important simplifying feature, since it means that one does not need a given therapeutic rule of thumb or recipe for diarrhea, another for pyloric stenosis, and still others for all of the many other types of specific clinical disorders that may be encountered in pediatric practice.

*Magnitude of deficits*
Much work has been done, the results of which allow an approximate quantitative picture of the magnitudes of deficits encountered in various disorders of hydration. The data obtained serve as average figures to be used as guides for replacement therapy as well as to provide a base of reference for analysis of the physiologic consequences of the losses. The soundest base of reference for conceptualizing deficits is *body weight*, since body stores of water and electrolytes are more closely proportional to body weight than to body surface area, caloric expenditure, and other variables.

Table 9 shows reasonable ranges of values estimated from data in the literature for three different types of dehydration in infants—so-called isotonic dehydration, in which plasma sodium concentration is normal or nearly normal (130 to 150 mEq/L); for hypertonic dehydration, in which the plasma sodium concentration is elevated (greater than 150 mEq/L); and for hypotonic dehydration, in which the initial plasma sodium is less than 130 mEq/L. In all cases, the degree of dehydration would be classified as moderate or severe.

Several features of these data are noteworthy. First, moderate or severe degrees of isotonic dehydration, in infants at least, are associated with loss of 10 to 15 percent of the body weight as water (100 to 150 ml/kg body weight). Second, appreciable sodium deficits are present and, in most instances, there is an approximately equal deficit of potassium as well. In other words, the deficits of cations are shared to an approximately equal extent by sodium and potassium. Third, the cation losses of sodium and potassium must be matched by some combination of the univalent anions chloride and bicarbonate, the exact proportion of each anion determined by the nature of the disease process. In pyloric stenosis, for example, losses of chloride are much greater than losses of bicarbonate, since the primary loss is hydrochloric acid from the stomach. In diarrhea, however, bicarbonate losses predominate over chloride relative to their normal relationship in plasma; hence, the patient develops a metabolic acidosis owing to bicarbonate loss. Clearly, the nature of the distribution of anion loss between chloride and bicarbonate determines the acid-base disturbance that will be manifested in the patient. Fourth, the nature of the loss of all ions in relation to the magnitude of water loss determines the osmolarity of the remaining body fluids. The virtual osmolarity of the loss can be calculated by dividing the sum of the amounts of sodium, potassium, and anions lost by the volume of the water loss. For example, in isotonic dehydration, the osmolarity of the loss is close to the normal value for plasma (280 mOsm/L). In hypertonic dehydration, the osmolarity of the loss is distinctly less than the normal value, whereas in hypotonic dehydration it is greater.

It should be emphasized that the loss, in essence, represents the *net negative balances* that have occurred over the period of illness prior to therapy and, therefore, takes account of all routes of loss and all routes of intake that the patient may have sustained, both normal and abnormal, prior to admission to the hospital. Thus, although diarrhea is typically associated with losses of hypotonic stool water, this is but one of several routes of loss that the patient may sustain, others being insensible water loss, sweat, and urine. Furthermore, some oral intake, usually of uncertain volume and composition, may have also occurred so that the loss of water or electrolyte may have been partially offset by this intake. Thus, although we are never in the position of ascertaining the exact magnitude of each component of the balance during the development of the illness, we can confidently assume that the net result of all components of the balance has been such as to result in an isotonic loss if the patient presents with dehydration and a normal plasma normal plasma sodium concentration. Similarly, a high initial plasma sodium concentration indicates that the net loss has been hypotonic, whereas a low initial plasma sodium concentration indicates that the net loss has been hypertonic.

### Effects of losses of water and electrolyte on the body fluids

It is important to understand the effects of the deficits of water and electrolyte on the composition of the remaining body fluids. This section will deal with the quantitative effects of losses of water and electrolyte in various proportions on the body fluids.

In this discussion, we will start with a normal TBW of 0.65 L/kg, a normal ECF of 0.25 L/kg, a normal ICF of 0.40 L/kg, and a normal osmolarity of 280 mOsm/L (i.e., two times the normal plasma sodium concentration). In each analysis, the assumption is made that the total cation loss is equally shared by sodium and potassium, but the anion losses are assumed to be chloride and bicarbonate. Varying proportions of the anion losses will not be specifically treated, since their distribution depends upon the specific nature of the loss and, thus, the resulting acid-base disorder. The fundamental assumptions underlying the analysis that follows are based upon the physiologic considerations that have been summarized earlier with respect to the well-established osmotic behavior of the body fluids.

*Isotonic dehydration* will be considered first. According to the considerations discussed earlier, the loss has been isotonic and has consisted of equal contributions of sodium and potassium (matched with chloride plus bicarbonate). Figure 25 shows a quantitative treatment of the effects of this type of loss in a patient who has sustained a loss of 100 ml/kg of body weight. The following are the major points of importance: (1) the total water deficit has been sustained entirely at the expense of the volume of the ECF; this is because the loss has been isotonic, thus leaving the body fluids isotonic, and therefore, no osmotic gradient has been generated and no internal redistribution of water has occurred, and (2) the ECF has "lost" a total of 14 mEq/kg of sodium, only half of which has been lost to the environment, the other half being "lost" to the ICF in exchange for potassium that has traversed the ECF and has been lost to the environment.

In this example, the ECF volume has been reduced by 40 percent (from 0.25 L/kg to 0.15 L/kg) and this in turn has major physiologic consequences. These arise principally because the

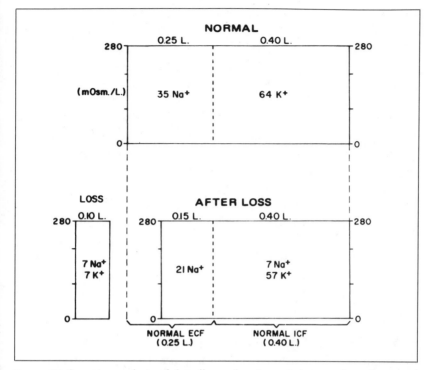

FIGURE 25. Stepwise analysis of the effects of an isotonic loss on the volume and composition of the body fluids of an infant. The upper diagram shows the volumes per kg of body weight of TBW, ECF, and ICF in a normal infant plotted on the horizontal axis. The osmolarity (i.e., 2 × plasma [Na$^+$]) is shown on the vertical axis. The numbers in the boxes representing ECF and ICF are the approximate content of ions in each space.

The lower diagram shows the effects of a loss from the ECF of 0.10 L/kg of water containing 7 mEq/kg of Na$^+$, 7 mEq/kg of K$^+$, and 14 mEq/kg of Cl$^-$ and HCO$_3^-$. The 7 mEq/kg of K$^+$ lost originated from the ICF; to preserve electroneutrality, an additional 7 mEg/kg of extracellular Na$^+$ has moved into the ICF. The amount of K$^+$ in the ICF has therefore fallen from 64 mEq/kg to 57 mEq/kg owing to the loss of 7 mEq/kg. The total amount of Na$^+$ in the ECF has been diminished by 14 mEq/kg—7 mEq/kg of which were lost to the environment and another 7 mEq/kg of which have been lost to the ICF. The volume of the ECF is now 0.15 L/kg. The final osmolarity is the same as the control; therefore, the final volume of ICF is unchanged—i.e., 0.40 L/kg.

plasma volume, which is an integral part of the ECF, participates to a nearly proportional extent in the contraction. This marked reduction in plasma volume in turn has serious consequences in terms of the maintenance of an intact circulation of blood. The resulting condition is not unlike that seen in hemorrhage, except that in dehydration, red blood cells are not lost; only the water and electrolyte content of the plasma is lost. This condition has been aptly termed the "white hemorrhage" since blood volume is reduced owing to the reduction of plasma volume, but no erythrocytes are lost. But in either the white or the red hemorrhage, a reduction in blood volume is accompanied initially by a reduction in the circulation of blood to skin and muscle, viscera, and later to the kidneys. With more severe degrees of reduction of plasma and blood volume, the circulation may be further compromised so that reversible and, eventually, irreversible shock supervenes. Indeed, it is shock that kills patients with dehydration, and the recognition of this fact is of paramount importance in therapy.

Both hypertonic and hypotonic dehydration may be analyzed in the same way as isotonic dehydration. Comparative quantitative sequences are summarized in Figures 26 and 27. *Hypertonic dehydration* (Figure 27) involves proportionately less severe reduction in ECF volume than does the same degree of isotonic dehydration (see Figure 25). This is because the elevated osmolarity of the ECF causes water to move from the ICF to the ECF. Thus, the ECF, although contracted, is less likely to be severely compromised than is the case with a comparable degree of isotonic dehydration. In view of this, it is not surprising that circulation is better maintained in hypertonic dehydration, and shock is relatively rare. Further, the usual signs of dehydration that are largely related to the degree of contraction of the ECF are typically less severe for any given degree of dehydration than is the case in isotonic dehydration. The opposite is true in *hypotonic dehydration* (compare Figures 25 and 26) in which the ECF water is not only lost to the environment, but an additional increment is osmotically transferred into the cells. It is not surprising that shock is much more likely to occur in hypotonic dehydration.

The changes in the volume of the ICF in the three types of dehydration are also worth noting. In isotonic dehydration, no change occurs in the volume of the ICF since there are no osmotic gradients produced. In hypertonic dehydration, the volume of the ICF diminishes; in hypotonic dehydration it increases. These changes do, in fact, occur in most tissue cells. But there is at least one type of cell that probably does not behave in this way, and this is the erythrocyte. If exposed acutely to a change in external sodium concentration, erythrocytes shrink or swell in a predictable manner. But if the abnormal osmotic environment is maintained for any appreciable length of time (probably some hours or even a day or more), the available evidence seems to indicate that the cell readjusts to a normal volume through a readjustment of intra-

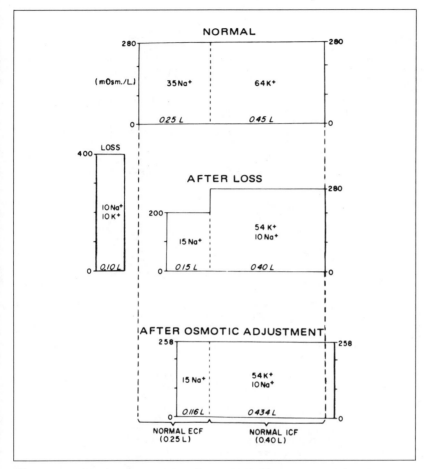

FIGURE 26. Stepwise analysis of the effects of a hypertonic loss on the volume and composition of the body fluids of an infant. The normal conditions are the same as those shown in Figure 27. The middle diagram indicates the initial effect of the loss on the ECF *before* any osmotic shifts of water have occurred; the lower diagram illustrates the new final steady state.

The loss is hypertonic, having a volume of 0.10 L/kg containing 10 mEq/kg each of $Na^+$ and $K^+$, and 20 mEq/kg of $Cl^-$ plus $HCO_3^-$. The osmolarity of the loss is therefore 400 mOsm/L. The immediate effect of the loss is to cause the ECF volume to be reduced by 0.10 L/kg and markedly hypotonic with an osmolarity of 200 mOsm/L. The ICF osmolarity is, however, 280 mOsm/L, and water movement now occurs such that the ECF volume of 0.15 L/kg is further reduced to a new final value of 0.116 L/kg; the ICF volume increases from 0.40 L/kg to 0.434 L/kg. The new final osmolarity is again equal in both compartments at a value of 258 mOsm/L, and the new plasma $[Na^+]$ is 129 mEq/L.

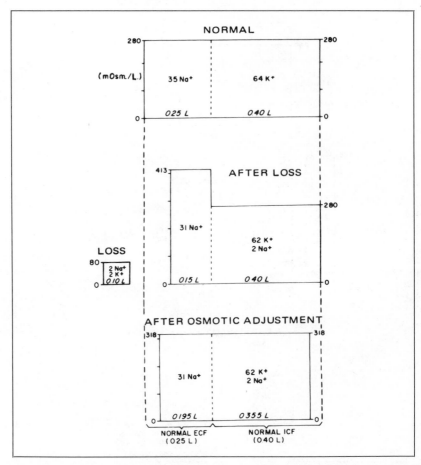

FIGURE 27. Stepwise analysis of the effects of a hypotonic loss on the volume and composition of the body fluids of an infant. The normal conditions are the same as shown in Figure 25. The middle diagram indicates the initial effect of the loss on the ECF *before* any osmotic shifts of water have occurred; the lower diagram shows the new final steady state.

The loss is hypotonic, having a volume of 0.10 L/kg of water containing 2 mEq/kg each of $Na^+$ and $K^+$ and 4 mEq/kg of $Cl^-$ plus $HCO_3^-$. The osmolarity of the loss is therefore 80 mOsm/L. The immediate effect of the loss is to cause the ECF volume to be reduced by 0.10 L/kg and markedly hypertonic with an osmolarity of 413 mOsm/L. The ICF osmolarity is, however, 280 mOsm/kg, and water movement now occurs such that the ECF volume of 0.15 L/kg is increased to a new final value of 0.195 L/kg; the ICF correspondingly decreases from 0.40 L/kg to 0.355 L/kg. The new final osmolarity is again equal in both compartments at a value of 318 mOsm/L, and the new plasma $[Na^+]$ is 159 mEq/L.

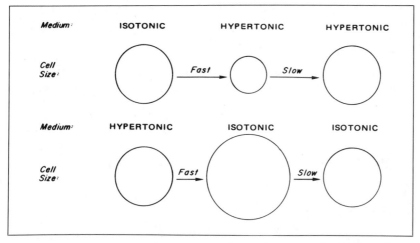

FIGURE 28. Postulated osmotic behavior of the erythrocyte with abrupt and sustained changes in extracellular osmolarity. The normal erythrocyte abruptly exposed to a hypertonic environment shows a rapid osmotic shift of water resulting in a reduction of cell volume. However, with time, intracellular solute is readjusted so that the cell swells to normal size. When such a readjusted cell is exposed abruptly to a normal osmotic environment, it swells to supernormal size; slow readjustment of intracellular solute follows to restore cell volume to normal.

cellular potassium content. This slow readjustment thus restores cell volume to normal in the face of a sustained abnormal osmotic environment. This sequence is depicted diagrammatically in Figure 28. If the abnormal osmotic environment is now abruptly readjusted to normal, the cell behaves acutely as though it were a perfect osmometer in that the cell volume that was previously readjusted to normal in the face of the sustained hypertonic environment, now swells as the cell is abruptly exposed to a normal osmotic environment. This can be readily detected by the usual osmotic fragility test. If this new normal osmotic environment is maintained, a slow readjustment occurs again by readjustment of intracellular potassium such that cell volume is again restored to normal.

It is possible that this peculiar behavior of the erythrocyte is also shared by neurons but probably not by muscle or other tissue cells (which comprise the bulk of the total ICF). This (assumed) peculiar osmotic behavior of neurons could be of considerable clinical importance, since it implies that any abrupt correction of hypertonic dehydration would be accompanied by a swelling of neurons to supernormal size, and this in turn may cause a variety of neurologic disorders during correction—most notably, convulsions.

This complication will be discussed further in the context of hypertonic dehydration.

*Formulation of replacement therapy for deficits*

In approaching a patient with dehydration, five key questions must be answered in order to formulate physiologically appropriate therapy. These questions are as follows:

1. What is the magnitude or degree of dehydration? Is it mild, moderate, or severe?
2. What is the type of dehydration present? Is it hypotonic, isotonic, or hypertonic?
3. Is a deficit of body potassium likely? If so, what is its approximate magnitude?
4. Is an acid-base disturbance present? If so, what type and how severe is it?
5. Is there any underlying nutritional deficit? If so, how severe is it?

Three sources of information are available to answer these questions: (1) the history of the patient, (2) the physical findings manifested by the patient, and (3) the data obtained by laboratory examination of the blood and the urine.

## ASSESSMENT OF THE MAGNITUDE OF DEHYDRATION

*Physical signs and history*

Theoretically, the deficits of water should be the difference between the measured values for TBW and ECF volume of any given patient and the normal values expected for that patient. In practice, however, the techniques used for such determinations are such as to preclude this approach in clinical medicine. Rather, the clinician must make a semiquantitative estimate of the magnitude of loss of body water using data derived from the history and the physical examination. In making this assessment, it is useful to bear in mind that there are approximate upper limits to the magnitude of an acute contraction of TBW and ECF that are compatible with life. Thus, in acute isotonic dehydration in infants, the upper limit of loss of total body water that is still compatible with life is about 15 percent of the body weight (i.e., 0.15 L/kg body weight). It should be recalled that in isotonic dehydration, this loss is sustained entirely by the ECF (see the preceding paragraphs).

The signs and symptoms of dehydration and, particularly, the circulatory changes of the dehydrated state correlate better with the degree of reduction of volume of the ECF than with the degree of reduction of TBW. An infant presenting with an acute isotonic dehydration amounting to 15 percent of his body weight will likely have sustained an approximate loss of ECF volume to a value of about 0.10 L/kg from the normal value of 0.25 L/kg. Under these circumstances, shock is very likely to be present, since there is marked diminution in blood volume and, accordingly, a very poor circulation. Blood pressure may be only barely maintained in the normal range, or it may be frankly low. Tachycardia is present. The circulation to the skin, muscles, and kidneys (the last producing prerenal azotemia, as is discussed in the following paragraphs) is diminished. The skin mucous membranes are dry, and the skin has poor turgor; the anterior fontanelle, if patent, is greatly depressed. The state of the peripheral circulation, as judged by the warmth and color of the skin and by the rapidity of filling of the cutaneous capillary bed when blanched, should be assessed.

Ideally, one could assess with considerable precision the magnitude of loss of total body water in such a patient by comparing a recent accurate pre-illness body weight with the body weight obtained on admission to the hospital. Pre-illness weights in infants are sometimes known by mothers as the result of recent well-baby visits. Suppose, for example, the infant is known to have weighed 4 kg shortly before the onset of diarrheal dehydration. After 3 days, the infant manifests severe dehydration and body weight is found to be 3.4 kg. The difference of 0.6 kg could be almost entirely attributable to the loss of body water and would amount to 0.15 L (0.6 kg/4.0 kg = 0.15 kg) of water lost per kilogram of initial body weight (i.e., 15% of initial body weight). Unfortunately, a recent accurate pre-illness weight is often not available; usually the clinician must evaluate the magnitude of dehydration from the severity of clinical signs and symptoms. The accurate serial measurement of the body weight on admission and at points during recovery from dehydration is probably the single most valuable measurement that can be made in assessing the initial state of the patient as well as the progress of therapy. It is regrettable that in most hospitals this most valuable measurement is carried out with little regard for obvious sources of error. Hence, in actual practice, the values for body weight often lack any meaning and may be frankly misleading, unless the measurements are given meticulous attention.

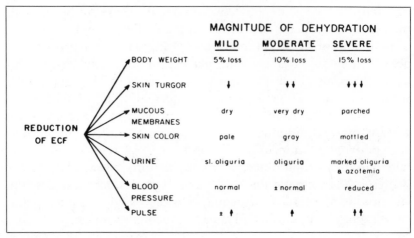

FIGURE 29. Changes expected as a result of increasing intensity of dehydration in the infant.

We have already seen that the degree of *severe* dehydration compatible with life is about 15 percent or 0.15 L/kg. *Moderate* degrees of dehydration are associated with losses of about 10 percent of initial body weight. Here the signs and symptoms of dehydration are present, but shock, although imminent, is not usually overt. Prerenal azotemia is likely to be present. *Mild* degrees of dehydration with equivocal signs of dehydration are associated with losses of approximately 5 percent of the body weight as water. Shock is absent in these cases, and prerenal azotemia is usually not present or is equivocal. Figure 29 depicts these three somewhat arbitrary stages of dehydration.

While admittedly approximate, these estimates of loss of body water and ECF are valuable in the initial formulation of therapy. This is not to say that continuing observation of the patient may not lead to an alteration of the initial estimate. The initial estimate, however, does provide a useful basis for the formulation of first step of therapy.

The *5–10–15 percent rule* (corresponding to mild, moderate, and severe degrees of dehydration) for assessment of the magnitude of isotonic dehydration applies to infants. In older children and in adults, the comparable figures are more likely to be 3 percent (mild), 6 percent (moderate), and 9 percent (severe). These differences between the infant and the older subject come about because the adult normally has a smaller TBW and a smaller ECF volume per kilogram of body weight than does the infant. Per kilogram of body weight, the adult who has lost 10 percent of his body weight as water from the ECF reduces the volume of the latter from the normal value of 0.20 L/kg to the new value of about 0.10 L/kg; whereas, the infant requires a 15 percent loss to cause his ECF volume to be reduced to the same level (from 0.25 L/kg to 0.10 L/kg). Thus, the infant can sustain proportionately greater losses than the adult before reaching the seemingly critical level of ECF volume for survival, which appears to be about 0.10 L/kg in both cases. However, due to the proportionately faster metabolic rate, the infant is likely to reach this lower limit at a faster rate than would the adult. In current practice, severe dehydration is very uncommon in adults in this country, whereas it still may be seen in infants; adults are likely to seek medical care at a relatively earlier stage in their longer course of development of dehydration since they are able to communicate clearly with others.

In assessing the magnitude of dehydration in the patient with hypertonic dehydration, it should be recalled that the ECF is relatively well maintained owing to the osmotic shift of water from intracellular to extracellular fluid (see Figure 26). In hypotonic dehydration, on the other hand, the losses to the environment are augmented by further osmotic transfers of water from extracellular to intracellular fluid (Figure 27). Thus, given the same degree of total water loss, the hypertonically dehydrated infant with a loss of 10 percent of body weight will have a proportionately greater ECF volume than the isotonically dehydrated infant. Conversely, the ECF volume is most vulnerable in hypotonic dehydration, and in this condition an infant will show more marked signs and symptoms than in isotonic dehydration of comparable magnitude. Estimates for each of these states are given in Table 9, and they may be used in appropriate cases.

*Laboratory data*
In general, laboratory data are of limited assistance in assessing the magnitude of dehydration. Obviously, with marked contraction of the ECF volume and the plasma volume, one might expect the erythrocytes and plasma proteins to be concentrated (so-called hemoconcentration) and the magnitude of this concentration to be related to the degree of contraction of the ECF. Although this phenomenon does occur, it cannot be used in practice in any precise way to estimate the degree of contraction present; accurate pre-illness values are never known, and any rise in the concentration of plasma proteins causes the ECF to be redistributed so

plasma volume is relatively increased at the expense of the ISF, owing to the increased colloidal osmotic pressure exerted by the proteins, which are confined to the plasma volume. For these reasons, the degree of hemoconcentration is not of any great quantitative value in infants although the presence of unequivocally high values for packed-cell volume or plasma proteins certainly confirms a clinical impression of marked dehydration.

Another chemical abnormality that confirms the presence of dehydration is prerenal azotemia. Prerenal azotemia occurs because of a compensatory renal circulatory adjustment incident to the reduction of plasma volume whereby renal blood flow falls. This fall is accompanied by a fall in glomerular filtration rate and, therefore, in urea clearance. Under all conditions, the concentration of urea in the body fluids is a function of the rate of urea production compared to the rate of urea excretion. Thus, a previously healthy patient may respond to short-term illness by a rather marked catabolism of endogenous body protein with a relatively large production of urea. If urea clearance is reduced in this patient, the blood urea nitrogen (BUN) may rise rather rapidly (Figure 30). Similarly, a continuing intake of protein in the face of reduction in glomerular filtration rate will raise the BUN rather rapidly. On the other hand, a protein-depleted patient whose urea production is low will have a much smaller rise in BUN in response to the same reduction in urea clearance and degree of dehydration. Thus, the magnitude of prerenal azotemia does not necessarily correlate with the magnitude of dehydration even though the occurrence of azotemia certainly indicates that a significant degree of dehydration is present, assuming renal disease can be excluded.

The plasma creatinine concentration, which is basically related to muscle mass, is theoretically more helpful in the detection of prerenal azotemia than is the blood urea nitrogen because it is less affected by the exogenous intake. However, it is often a difficult measurement to make accurately in most laboratories, and, furthermore, infants characteristically have relatively small amounts of muscle mass. Thus, the normal plasma creatinine concentration in infants is approximately one third of the adult values. Because of these factors, the measurement of plasma creatinine concentration as it is usually performed is often not a reliable, practical indicator of prerenal azotemia, even though in theory it should be. On the other hand, if one is confident of the accuracy of the measurement and aware of the relatively low normal concentrations

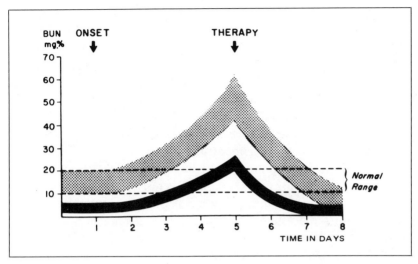

FIGURE 30. Prerenal azotemia in dehydration. The approximate time course is indicated for the development of prerenal azotemia during dehydration in a subject with previously normal protein stores (*dotted zone*). The onset of therapy is accompanied by a marked reduction in the blood urea nitrogen (*BUN*) to or below the normal range. The black zone indicates the probable time relationships for the development of prerenal azotemia in a subject who was previously protein depleted. The "normal" values for such a subject would be lower than the usually accepted normal range; the BUN, with dehydration, may not rise above the usually accepted normal range because the rate of production of urea by such protein-depleted subjects is low.

usually present in infants, the measurement can be of considerable value.

Examination of the urine should be carried out on all patients with dehydration, and the findings from a routine urinalysis should, in general, be consistent with the diagnosis of dehydration. Dehydration imposes a demand on the kidney to conserve water. Accordingly, the urine should be concentrated, with a specific gravity usually greater than 1.020. The urine may often contain traces of protein and a few formed elements, these being attributable probably to secondary renal circulatory changes. A dilute urine in the face of dehydration suggests that a defect in the urinary concentration mechanism is present (owing perhaps to pituitary or nephrogenic diabetes insipidus when the specific gravity is generally less than 1.010 or to intrinsic renal disease with the specific gravity being fixed in the range of 1.010 to 1.012). Potassium depletion of long standing may lead to a urinary concentrating defect as part of the potassium deficiency nephropathy. Large volumes of urine are passed in dehydrated patients undergoing solute diuresis, the most important example being diabetic glycosuria.

Sodium depletion likewise imposes maximal stimuli for renal conservation of sodium, so, ordinarily, the urine of a salt-depleted, dehydrated subject is virtually free of sodium. However, it should be recalled that in several disorders, renal salt-wasting may be present—for example, owing to diuretics, intrinsic renal disease, or to extrarenal (e.g., adrenocortical) disease. Under these conditions, the urinary sodium should be measured. Although a 24-hour measurement for urinary sodium is most desirable (especially when the intake of sodium is low), it is often not feasible to withhold sodium replacement therapy for such a long period of time in order to collect the specimen from the patient in the untreated state. A practical diagnostic shortcut consists of measuring the urinary sodium concentration on a casual specimen of urine prior to instituting therapy. In general, a significant salt loss via the urine will be manifested by a urinary sodium concentration on such a specimen of at least 60 mEq/L, and often it is much higher. In general, however, urinary sodium concentration on a casual sample under rapidly changing intakes of sodium can be very deceptive unless it is very low (a few mEq/L) or very high (80 or more mEq/L).

## CLASSIFICATION OF THE TYPE OF DEHYDRATION

Whereas the estimate of the degree of dehydration in any given patient is at best an educated guess, the type of dehydration can be determined with great precision through the measurement of the initial sodium concentration of the plasma. Thus, if the sodium concentration is within the general range of 130 to 150 mEq/L, the dehydration is classified as *isotonic*, or essentially so. If the initial sodium concentration exceeds 150 mEq/L, the dehydration is classified as *hypertonic*, and values less than 130 mEq/L are associated with *hypotonic* dehydration.

There are a few physical signs pointing specifically towards hypertonic dehydration, especially in infants. Most important of these is the "doughlike" feel of the skin. Areas of sclerema may appear, particularly around the buttocks and thighs. Disturbances of consciousness—coma or semicoma—are frequently encountered in severely hypernatremic infants. Severe hypotonic dehydration is not accompanied by any specific physical signs; its presence

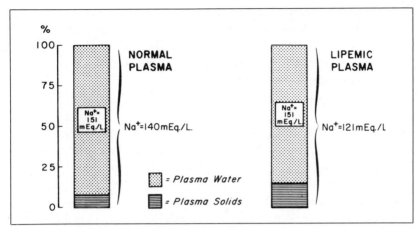

FIGURE 31. Hyponatremia as an artifact secondary to hyperlipemia. The bar on the left shows the composition of normal plasma in terms of plasma water (93%) and plasma solids, largely protein (7%). Solutes such as sodium are dissolved only in the plasma water, making a concentration of sodium in the plasma water of 151 mEq/L. The bar on the right shows the effects of increasing the plasma solids by increasing the lipids, with a commensurate reduction in the amount of water present per liter of plasma. Thus, although the sodium concentration per liter of plasma may be low, the sodium concentration per liter of plasma water may be normal.

is suggested by severe or unexpected peripheral vascular collapse in a patient whose history does not suggest severe extrarenal loss. The signs of water intoxication owing to acute swelling of brain cells do not usually occur in hypotonic dehydration, perhaps because the hypotonic state has developed over an interval long enough to permit readjustment of neuronal cell volume.

Although certain signs and symptoms and certain disease processes may point to the occurrence of hypertonic or hypotonic dehydration, the ultimate means of identifying the type of dehydration requires the measurement and interpretation of the plasma sodium concentration. There are two possible situations in which the plasma sodium concentration will not accurately reflect the osmolarity of the body fluids. One of these is the so-called hyponatremia due to hyperlipemia. Normally, the plasma consists of about 93 percent water and 7 percent solids, of which plasma proteins are the most important. The electrolytes of the plasma are dissolved only in the water phase; therefore, with the normal sodium concentration in plasma of 140 mEq/L, the concentration of sodium in the *plasma water* would be 140 mEq/0.93L = 151 mEq/L of plasma water (Figure 31). It is this concentration of sodium that most closely approximates that of the ISF, since proteins do not cross the capillary membrane to any appreciable extent. As long as the ratio of plasma water to plasma solids is not greatly altered, as is the case in most diseases, there is a very close relationship between the concentration of sodium in the plasma and the concentration of sodium in the plasma water.

In grossly lipemic plasma, however, the lipids, being anhydrous, accumulate, and the concentration of plasma solids increases per liter of plasma. The fraction of plasma water in the plasma, thus, falls. Hence, although the sodium concentration in the *plasma water* may still be normal at 151 mEq/L, the sodium concentration *per liter of plasma* is reduced, because one liter of plasma now contains less water and more solids (see Figure 31). Recognition of this type of hyponatremia is relatively straightforward since the plasma will be milky owing to its high lipid content. The same type of effect has been reported in rare macroglobulinemic states as well. Measurement of either plasma water content or plasma osmolarity will detect this effect.

Somewhat more frequently, "artifactual" hyponatremia occurs when there is concomitant *hyperglycemia* as in uncontrolled diabetes. Glucose behaves as a poorly permeating solute in that it does not readily enter cells, particularly in the absence of insulin. Being largely excluded from cells, it behaves as an osmotically active particle and causes water to shift from the intracellular to the extracellular fluid. This water movement in turn dilutes all extracellular solutes, of which sodium is the most important. The osmolarity contributed by glucose can be readily calculated from the measured plasma sugar concentration. Recall that the molecular weight of glucose is 180; therefore, 1 mM of glucose equals one milliosmole (mOsm). Suppose a diabetic patient has a blood sugar of 900 mg/100 ml (equivalent to 9000 mg/L) and a plasma sodium concentration of 115 mEq/L. The sodium concentration alone suggests hypotonic dehydration. However, one must also consider the osmotic effect of glucose:

$$\text{mOsm from glucose} = \frac{9000 \text{ mg/L}}{180 \text{ mg/mM}} = 50 \text{ mOsm/L}$$

Thus, the osmolarity contributed by electrolytes is twice the plasma sodium concentration ($2 \times 115$ mEq/L or 230 mOsm/L), but with the added 50 mOsm/L from glucose, the effective osmolarity of the plasma is 280 mOsm—an isotonic value. In such patients, reduction of the blood sugar (e.g., with insulin therapy) causes water to move back into cells, and the plasma sodium concentration will rise accordingly.

## THE RECOGNITION OF POTASSIUM DEFICITS

Published data show that potassium as well as sodium is generally lost from the body in most types of dehydration, whether dehydration is due to diarrhea, pyloric stenosis, gastrointestinal fistula drainage, or other causes (see Table 9). Indeed, it is usually a safe assumption that some degree of potassium depletion is present when, as in these disorders, there has been a poor intake coupled with an appreciable loss of gastrointestinal fluids. However, the potassium depletion occurs not only from a direct loss in the gastrointestinal fluids but also from losses in the urine as a part of the early renal response to the acid-base disorders that nearly always accompany these disturbances. In diabetic acidosis, this early renal response involving an augmented excretion of potassium (prior to the achievement of maximal ammonium production) is probably the principal route by which potassium is lost. This may be exacerbated by losses of potassium caused by vomiting, which often accompanies this disorder, and, of course, the vomiting also precludes any oral replacement. It is safest to assume that some potassium deficit accompanies all forms of dehydration with very few exceptions, these being simple water deprivation, diabetes insipidus, adrenocortical insufficiency, and greatly advanced renal disease.

Body potassium depletion may be present even in the absence of hypokalemia, as has been discussed already (see Figure 19). Indeed, the initial plasma potassium value may be normal or elevated, particularly in acidotic patients or in patients with prerenal azotemia, even though the body stores of potassium are reduced. For example, a diabetic in severe acidosis may have a plasma potassium concentration between 5 and 6 mEq/L. However, as the acidosis and dehydration are corrected, the plasma potassium concentration often falls precipitously to frankly hypokalemic values, thus more accurately reflecting the true state of the body stores of potassium (Figure 19).

## THE DIAGNOSIS OF ACID-BASE DISORDERS

The diagnosis of any acid-base disturbance, whether or not it coexists with a disorder of hydration, requires two types of fundamental information. (1) clinical information, which basically identifies the presence of a disorder known to produce an abnormal gain or loss of acid, base of $CO_2$ from the body, and (2) chemical information that documents a characteristic pattern of displacement of blood acid-base equilibrium consistent with the type of acid-base disturbance produced by the particular clinical disorder present. The various etiologic factors underlying the development of acid-base disorders and the characteristic changes in the blood that are encountered in these disorders are summarized in Tables 2 and 3. To diagnose metabolic acidosis, for example, one must identify the presence of a specific disease process known to produce a gain of strong acid (e.g., diabetes) or a loss of bicarbonate from the ECF (e.g., diarrhea). Metabolic acidosis is then confirmed by the finding of a low plasma bicarbonate concentration (reflecting the primary abnormality), a low plasma $PCO_2$ (signifying respiratory compensation), and a low blood pH. Even in the absence of measurement of blood pH and $PCO_2$, a low value for plasma bicarbonate concentration strongly confirms the impression of a metabolic acidosis, although not with as high a degree of confidence as would a complete chemical characterization of the acid-base status of blood (i.e., measurement of blood pH, plasma $PCO_2$, and plasma bicarbonate concentration). Furthermore, the anion pattern of the plasma and, in particular, the relationship between plasma chloride and undetermined anion fraction (see the following paragraphs) should be consistent with the underlying etiology of the acid-base disorder.

## Undetermined anion fraction

There is a simple but very useful method for evaluating changes in the *undetermined anion* (UA) fraction of the plasma. Close inspection of the normal plasma cation-anion pattern plotted (see Figure 3) as a "Gamblegram" (after the late Dr. James Gamble) reveals that the sum of the positive charges contributed by calcium, magnesium, and potassium (about 12 mEq/L) approximates the negative charge contributed by proteinate (about 15 mEq/L). If the small difference between these two is assumed to be insignificant, the UA fraction, sometimes called the *anion gap*, can be approximated by calculating the difference between the plasma sodium concentration and the sum of the concentrations of plasma chloride and bicarbonate:

$$\text{Anion gap} = ([Na^+]) - ([HCO_3^-] + [Cl^-])$$

In normal plasma, the anion gap usually averages 10 to 15 mEq/L in both adults and infants, depending in part on the individual laboratory's normal values and in part on whether arterial or venous blood is being used. The total $CO_2$ content can be used in lieu of bicarbonate concentration without any significant difference in the final result.

Some authors define the anion gap as $([Na^+] + [K^+]) - ([HCO_3^-] + [Cl^-])$. With this information, the anion gap will have slightly different values for normal, but it will serve the same purposes that are discussed in the text. There is sometimes a tendency to overinterpret the anion gap. One must remember that it represents a small difference between two sets of large numbers, each of which has a finite analytic error. In general, an increase in the anion gap must be at least 5 mEq/L or so *above* the usual normal value to be regarded as possibly significant. The anion gap is also useful in detecting laboratory errors, since it is very rare to encounter a disorder in which the anion gap is less than 5 mEq/L and virtually impossible for it to be zero or a negative value. If one encounters extremely low or negative values for the anion gap, one may assume that an error has been made in the laboratory determination of one of the components entering into the calculation of this fraction, and all determinations should be repeated.

It is apparent from the buffer reactions in Table 2 that the addition of any strong acid (other than hydrochloric acid) will cause an increase in the anion gap, since the anion $(X^-)$ of the loading acid $(H^+X^-)$ will appear in the undetermined anion fraction and will, thus, be reflected by a value for the anion gap above the normal value of 10 to 15 mEq/L. On the other hand, the anion gap tends to be in the normal range in uncomplicated hyperchloremic acidosis due to bicarbonate loss, as in diarrhea or renal tubular acidosis, as well as in the usual instances of respiratory acidosis and alkalosis and in metabolic alkalosis.

There is a tendency for the anion gap to increase somewhat when there is prerenal azotemia secondary to dehydration. This is due to the retention of phosphate, sulfate, and the other anions found in azotemic states. Such increases accompanying prerenal azotemia rarely exceed the normal value by more than about 5 mEq/L.

## ASSESSMENT OF NUTRITIONAL STATUS

The previous nutritional history and growth pattern of the patient plus simple anthropometric measurements (body weight, length or height, head circumference, and skin-fold thicknesses) form the first line of assessment of the nutritional status. To these measurements should be added certain routine chemical tests, notably plasma albumin and blood urea concentrations.

Proteins having shorter half-lives than albumin, such as prealbumin, retinol-binding protein, and others, are generally more useful in assessing a successful therapeutic regimen, since they are among the first to return to normal. But a sustained increase in body weight and a later increase in length (or height) as well as the return of the skin-fold thicknesses to or toward their respective normal levels are sure signs that restitution of lean body mass and fat are occurring.

It is beyond the scope of this book to discuss the more complex measures of nutritional assessment or to evaluate their usefulness. The important lesson is that serious nutritional disorders often underlie an acute disorder of hydration; once the disorder of hydration is successfully managed, the nutritional disorder must be assessed and also managed. Many special types of nutritional products for enteral use are available. In addition, safe and successful parenteral nutrition is now a reality, and given the appropriate indications, it may be an extremely useful modality in the management of the malnourished patient. This technique is discussed in detail in Chapter 5.

## SUMMARY OF ANALYSIS OF DEHYDRATION
Table 10 summarizes the five key questions that must be answered in formulating a therapeutic program for any patient with dehydration. The table also gives the most important sources of information for answering these questions.

## REPLACEMENT OF DEFICITS
### Chronological sequence of therapy of dehydration
The aim of all deficit therapy is to provide sufficient water, electrolyte, calories, and other nutritive requirements in reasonable amounts and in a sequence that will bring about an orderly and safe restoration of depleted body stores of all substances that have been lost. It is conceptually useful (Figure 32) to divide the deficit fluid program into four distinct, more or less arbitrary sequential phases:

> Phase I begins at the time of admission to the hospital and lasts 2 to 4 hr. During this time, therapy is aimed primarily at restoration of circulatory integrity.
> Phase II encompasses the next 18 to 24 hr (after admission). During this time, the primary aims are the partial restoration

TABLE 10. Sources of Information for Analysis of Dehydration

| Questions to be Answered | Sources of Information |
|---|---|
| Magnitude of dehydration | 1. Loss of body weight<br>2. Clinical estimate of severity<br>Severity in isotonic dehydration |

| Severity | Infants | Older children and adults |
|---|---|---|
| Mild | 50 ml/kg ( 5%) | 30 ml/kg (3%) |
| Moderate | 100 ml/kg (10%) | 60 ml/kg (6%) |
| Severe | 150 ml/kg (15%) | 90 ml/kg (9%) |

| Questions to be Answered | Sources of Information |
|---|---|
| Type of dehydration | 1. Pathophysiology of specific illness<br>2. Specific physical signs, if any<br>3. Measurement of initial plasma $[Na^+]$<br>    Isotonic: plasma $[Na^+]$ = 130–150 mEq/L<br>    Hypertonic: plasma $[Na^+]$ = >150 mEq/L<br>    Hypotonic: plasma $[Na^+]$ = <130 mEq/L |
| Presence of deficit of body potassium | 1. Pathophysiology of specific illness interpreted in the light of retention balance data<br>2. Measurement of plasma $[K^+]$, particularly after abnormal acid-base status is corrected |
| Nature of acid-base disturbance | 1. Pathophysiology of specific illness to indicate type of etiologic factor<br>2. Measurement of blood acid-base status<br>3. Expected changes in UA fraction |
| Presence and degree of nutritional deficit | 1. Anthropometric measurements<br>2. Measurement of short half-life proteins, albumin, and urea-N in plasma |

of extracellular sodium and water deficits and the partial correction of acid-base disturbances.

Phase III lasts 1 to 4 days. During this time, the aim is to restore body potassium deficits and to complete the restoration of ECF volume and acid-base equilibrium.

Phase IV may last from one to several weeks or even longer. During this time, the aim is to restore body stores of fat and protein previously lost as a result of the disorder.

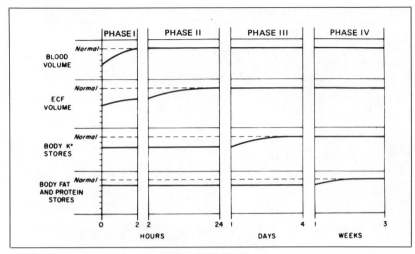

FIGURE 32. Chronologic sequence of therapy in dehydration, showing the idealized course of the four phases of fluid therapy in a patient with dehydration (see text). Maintenance therapy, normal and abnormal, must also be provided each day by the oral or parenteral route.

Since it is obvious that restoration of water, sodium, potassium, and acid or base deficits cannot be corrected instantaneously but, rather, will require several days, parenteral maintenance requirements—both normal and abnormal—must also be provided for each day of therapy.

There are sound physiologic reasons why the chronologic sequence of deficit therapy is appropriate. Shock, imminent or overt, is the greatest threat to life and requires the most urgent attention. In addition, restoration of the circulating blood volume will restore adequate renal function, which may have been impaired by dehydration and without which the fine adjustments necessary for accurate and complete restoration of normal volume and composition of the body fluids and its subdivisions are impossible. Once the circulation is adequately restored (phase I), further restoration of extracellular sodium and water deficits is undertaken (phase II). This also further bolsters the circulatory integrity and makes any ongoing losses less threatening. In addition, partial, usually substantial correction of the acid-base disorders ought to be achieved during phase II, thereby reducing the threat of severe acidosis or alkalosis. These goals are achieved by a combination of exogenous fluid therapy and, to a considerable extent, by restoration of renal corrective mechanisms incident to the expansion of the ECF and plasma volume.

Once the extracellular water and sodium deficits and the circulatory volume are largely restored, attention is directed to the repair of the body potassium stores (phase III). Although nearly all of the body potassium loss in typical dehydration will have been sustained at the expense of the intracellular potassium, this deficit can be replaced only via the ECF, in which the potassium concentration is normally very low relative to the normal concentration in the ICF. In order to avoid a transient and potentially dangerous degree of hyperkalemia during restoration, it is essential that body potassium stores be replaced over several days by continuous provision of small amounts of potassium, which in the aggregate will be sufficient to fully restore the deficit. Thus, sodium stores can usually be replaced safely in a matter of *hours*, but the time needed for safe replacement of the potassium deficit is a matter of *days*.

In uncomplicated instances, the patient is usually meeting some or even most fluid and electrolyte requirements by mouth during phase III. As improvement continues, substantial caloric and protein intakes can be offered and will be retained. Thus, the oral intake becomes the main route for the restoration of body fat and body protein stores during phase IV. In some instances, particularly in chronic protracted illnesses or in the presence of complications that interfere with an adequate oral intake of food, the parenteral route must be considered the main if not the sole channel for the provision of calories, nitrogen, and other requirements. Thus, despite adequate fluid and electrolyte replacement and good hydration, a continuous negative balance of calories and nitrogen may prove life threatening. In such cases, it is essential to provide adequate total parenteral nutrition. For this purpose, fluids containing amino acids, glucose, fat, and vitamins should be given. This topic is discussed in more detail in Chapter 5, Parenteral Nutrition.

## Feedback points during therapy

In any situation requiring fluid therapy, it is essential that therapy be planned step by step in accordance with general phases. See Figure 33, page 119 and Author's Notes 2, page 161. At the completion of each phase, systematic clinical and chemical reevaluation of the patient should be made. On the basis of feedback information, the adequacy of the previous therapeutic phase can be assessed and accurate plans for the next phase of therapy can be made.

Feedback information consists of two general types: (1) clinical information derived from the serial observation of the patient, and (2) chemical information derived from the repeated analyses of blood for the relevant constituents. On admission to the hospital, the admission examination should include an accurate determination of body weight, a careful assessment of the circulatory status (pulse rate, blood pressure, state of peripheral circulation, and other factors), evaluation of a timed urinary output (and, subsequently, an accurate record of water and electrolyte intake over given periods of time), and, finally, determination of the presence and intensity of the various signs of dehydration. Chemically, the electrolyte and acid-base composition of the blood or plasma should be determined as well as the hemoglobin concentration, hematocrit, plasma protein, and plasma total solids. Urinary specific gravity, semiquantitative tests for sugar and ketones, and urine pH provide additional points of information.

A summary of the types of feedback information and their timing is given in Table 11. Thus, at the end of Phase I the feedback information is largely clinical and consists of a reassessment of the circulation as judged by blood pressure and pulse rate as well as signs indicating adequacy of the circulatory status of the skin (color, warmth, and other factors). An increase in urine flow with a decrease in specific gravity indicates an augmented renal circulation. An improvement in state of consciousness likely signifies a significant increase in cerebral blood flow.

It is obvious that a fairly large number of variables are being followed in the feedback process, and unless these are well organized in the medical record, they may lose their effectiveness. At the time of admission, it is useful to lay out an organizational format of these data by lining off two blank sheets of paper, each showing time intervals in the far left-hand column. One sheet should be divided into columns, each column representing a particularly important clinical datum; comparable columns on the other sheet should be used for recording the observed chemical data. Once these data are organized and presented in this form, all important aspects of each phase of fluid therapy are immediately evident. It is the author's opinion that the designing of these summary sheets together with the diligent recording of all of the data constitutes one of the most useful teaching devices available for students who wish to master this field.

The second formal feedback point is at the end of phase II, during which time partial restoration of extracellular sodium and water deficits and partial correction of acid-base status are the

TABLE 11. Feedback Information During Fluid Therapy

| Therapeutic Phase | Feedback Information and Expected Changes |
|---|---|
| Phase I (0–4 hr); restoration of the circulation | 1. Improvement in circulatory signs (blood pressure, pulse, peripheral circulation)<br>2. Increase in urine flow<br>3. Improvement in state of consciousness |
| Phase II (2–24 hr); partial restoration of ECF deficit and acid-base status | 1. Gain of body weight<br>2. Sustained adequate urine flow<br>3. Stable adequate circulation<br>4. Decreased intensity of signs of dehydration<br>5. Partial or complete restoration of abnormal plasma [$Na^+$]<br>6. Fall in BUN to or toward normal<br>7. Partial restoration of abnormal blood acid-base status |
| Phase III (18 hr–4 days); restoration of body $K^+$ deficit | 1. Sustained gain in body weight<br>2. Normal of low BUN<br>3. Normal plasma [$Na^+$]<br>4. Normal acid-base status<br>5. Normal plasma [$K^+$] |
| Phase IV (2 days–3 wk); restoration of caloric and protein deficits | 1. Slow, steady gain in body weight<br>2. All plasma constituents normal |

major aims. An accurate body weighing at the end of phase II should reveal a substantial gain corresponding to one half to two thirds of the estimated total water deficit, depending upon the volume of fluid administered over Phases I and II and the estimated or measured output. Urinary flow should have been maintained at an adequate rate, and urinary specific gravity should be correspondingly dilute, indicating excretion of solutes in an adequate urinary volume. Stability of circulation should continue. At this point, remeasurement of the blood urea nitrogen and plasma creatinine concentrations should reveal substantial falls from previously elevated values to or toward normal. A partial or complete restoration of an initially abnormal plasma sodium concentration should have been accomplished. Remeasurement of the blood acid-base status should show a substantial correction toward normal.

Feedback information during phase III consists of accurate assessment of the patient's body weight serially, preferably on a daily basis. The pattern of satisfactory results is such that weight gained in the early phases of therapy is sustained, and smaller increments would not be registered. It should be emphasized that the accurate measurement of body weight is one of the most important variables in the assessment of successful management of the patient with dehydration. It is crucial in the quantitative formulation and assessment of the various phases of the fluid therapy program to be undertaken. Regrettably, the importance of this measurement is not appreciated in practice, and it is usually delegated to the lowest echelon of the nursing staff. Furthermore, the scales used are rarely calibrated, and the actual techniques do not take into account the weight of arm and leg boards, restraints, and other extraneous factors.

Blood urea nitrogen and plasma creatinine concentrations should now be normal or even low, since the patient is not yet on adequate protein intake and urea production is low. Accurate measurement of plasma creatinine concentration is preferable to measurement of BUN for the detection of prerenal azotemia, since it is much less dependent on the intake of protein, as was discussed earlier.

Plasma sodium concentration and blood acid-base status should achieve normal values during this period. In addition, if the restoration of body potassium deficits is proceeding at a satisfactory rate, the directional movement of plasma potassium concentration should be toward the normal limit.

Feedback information during phase IV, the period devoted to restoration of body mass, consists of a slower but steady regain of weight signifying deposition of new body fat and body tissue. Plasma electrolytes, acid-base status, blood urea nitrogen, and other requirements should be normal during this period. In addition to measurement of weight gain, repeated measurement of skin-fold thickness and plasma albumin concentration as well as, perhaps, plasma amino acid pattern may all be helpful in ascertaining nutritional status and recovery from a preexisting state of protein or caloric malnutrition.

## THERAPY OF PHASE I—RESTORATION OF THE CIRCULATION

The aim of the first phase of fluid therapy is to prevent imminent shock or to treat overt shock. Clearly, not all or even most patients with dehydration will necessarily require such specific therapy, since only severely dehydrated patients are likely to manifest serious circulatory problems. Furthermore, circulatory insufficiency requiring specific therapy for shock is relatively rare in hypertonic dehydration because the intracellular fluid has shared in the total water loss, and the extracellular fluid volume is relatively well maintained. However, in isotonic and to a greater degree in hypotonic dehydration, inadequacy of the circulation requiring specific therapy of the type discussed in the following paragraphs may be encountered; very occasionally this dehydration may be in a severe form.

In current practice in the United States, it is relatively uncommon to encounter a dehydrated patient with overt shock, probably because patients are referred earlier in the course of their illness. However, careful serial monitoring of the pulse rate and blood pressure of these patients will often show a pattern suggesting that there has been some degree of depletion of plasma volume.

In any individual patient the assessment of the adequacy of the circulation and determination of the need for specific therapy to bolster it is a clinical decision made at the time of the patient's admission to the hospital, based upon signs, symptoms, history, and other factors, as were discussed earlier. At this early point in the patient's course, no chemical data are available. Even if they were, they would not likely be of primary importance in deciding whether the circulatory dynamics were sufficiently impaired to require specific rapid correction.

### Theoretical considerations

Since shock is the most serious threat to life in dehydration, it deserves the highest priority in therapy. Theoretically, for the immediate purpose of rapid replacement of blood volume, one would use the fluid that, volume for volume, has the *smallest* volume of distribution within the body water. It follows that the ideal fluid for the therapy of shock secondary to dehydration would be that fluid that shows the least tendency to escape from the vascular compartment. The list of fluids in decreasing order of preference for the immediate purpose of expanding blood volume (i.e., the smallest to the largest volume of distribution) are: (1) packed erythrocytes or whole blood itself, (2) blood plasma or plasma expanders, (3) isotonic sodium-containing fluids, and (4) non–electrolyte-containing fluids, such as glucose in water.

Although the above theoretical analysis is sound, the order of priorities must be changed in order to cope with reality. Furthermore, one is not necessarily limited by the volume-for-volume argument on which the above considerations are based, since a greater volume of fluid than that lost can be administered. Although blood transfusion might be desirable, it takes time to obtain properly typed and cross-matched blood, and one does not wish to waste this time before treating a patient whose circulatory status is tenuous. However, with a patient suffering from overt shock, it is wise to obtain a blood sample on admission for typing and cross matching, since whole blood transfusion may be required later (see the discussion in the following paragraphs). Both whole blood and pooled plasma carry the risks of disseminating hepatitis, making their use undesirable.

## Initial hydrating infusion

In view of the considerations outlined, the therapy of phase I should usually consist of an initial hydrating infusion containing sodium in approximately isotonic proportions. Generally, in moderate dehydration the amount of such an initial hydrating infusion is about 10 ml/kg, and the rate of the infusion is generally about 5 ml/kg/hr for the first two or more hours comprising phase I. In overt shock, a rate of 10 or even more ml/kg/hr is needed, the exact rate depending upon continuing assessment of the response of the collapsed circulation. The intravenous route must always be used for all infusions regardless of the severity of dehydration, since it is only through this route that the fluid can actually be delivered directly into the circulation. The use of specifically designed pediatric intravenous needles and sets for this purpose makes this route feasible and preferable in skilled hands. If a superficial vein is not accessible, a cutdown and direct cannulation of an ankle vein is indicated and should be carried out.

It is risky to use any route other than the intravenous one in the therapy of covert or overt shock. Fluid introduced into the subcutaneous spaces or given by mouth will be absorbed slowly and irregularly, since blood flow through these areas is compromised as part of the compensatory circulatory adjustment incident to the general reduction of blood volume.

TABLE 12. Electrolyte Composition of Initial Hydrating Infusions

|  | Water (ml) | Na$^+$ (mEq) | Cl$^+$ (mEq) | HCO$_3$$^-$ (mEq) |
|---|---|---|---|---|
| Isotonic saline |  |  |  |  |
| Normal saline 0.9% | 1000 | 154 | 154 | 0 |
| Extracellular replacement fluid |  |  |  |  |
| Mixture for 1 liter |  |  |  |  |
| Normal saline, 0.9% | 844 | 130 | 130 | 0 |
| Sodium bicarbonate (1 mEq/ml) | 24 | 24 | 0 | 24 |
| Dextrose 5% in water (q.s. to make 1 liter) | 132 | 0 | 0 | 0 |
| Total | 1000 | 154 | 130 | 24 |

In general, one of two fluids should be used for the initial hydrating infusion: (1) isotonic saline (i.e., sodium chloride, 0.9%) containing 154 mEq/L of sodium and 154 mEq/L of chloride, and (2) an isotonic solution containing 154 mEq/L sodium, with the anions adjusted to contain 25 to 40 mEq/L of bicarbonate or bicarbonate-precursor and the remainder being chloride. (Solutions of this type will be referred to as *ECF replacement fluids.* See Table 16.) Reference is made to the section on the mixing of intravenous solutions (see p. 148). An example of a tailor-made ECF replacement solution is shown in Table 12.

Isotonic saline is the fluid of choice for patients suspected of having a metabolic alkalosis (or respiratory alkalosis), whereas one of the ECF replacement fluids is the choice for patients with dehydration and metabolic acidosis (or respiratory acidosis). The difference between these fluids is, of course, the absence or presence of the anion, bicarbonate (or bicarbonate-precursor). Infusion of a nonbicarbonate-containing fluid in a patient with metabolic acidosis—for example, infantile diarrhea—would induce a dilution acidosis that would make the acid-base status of the patient even more tenuous than it already is. For example, consider an infant with diarrheal acidosis and severe dehydration with a plasma bicarbonate concentration of 4.5 mEq/L and a plasma PCO$_2$ of 15 mm Hg. Even with this degree of respiratory compensation, blood pH would be very low (pH 7.10). Were this infant to receive a large initial hydrating infusion of isotonic saline (e.g., 20 to 30 ml/kg) in the course of treating shock in phase I, there would be a theoretical dilution of the already low plasma bicarbonate concentration by 20–30 percent, a reduction that even with the same level of respiratory compensation would cause a further fall in blood pH to levels of 7.0 or below—hardly a desirable effect in a patient having a very serious degree of acidemia prior to therapy. It is exactly in this situation—the presence of a severe contraction of extracellular fluid coupled with a severe acidemia—that dilution acidosis produced by a rapid infusion of normal saline, is most likely to occur.

This problem can be readily avoided; indeed, the acidosis may be relieved by the use of an ECF replacement fluid. Use of such a fluid would seem to be logical and preferable for such a patient.

Of the ECF replacement group, fluids containing bicarbonate-precursors such as acetate, lactate, or gluconate have often been used in place of a bicarbonate-containing fluid. These fluids are quite satisfactory if one can be assured that the bicarbonate precursor will in fact be metabolized to bicarbonate. The metabolism of such substances, however, is likely to be limited by the ability of the circulation to deliver the bicarbonate-precursor (plus oxygen) to the site of metabolism of the precursor to bicarbonate; this may be precisely where the problem lies in patients, particularly infants, with dehydration and imminent or overt circulatory collapse. If the bicarbonate-precursors are not metabolized, they of course cannot produce bicarbonate. Rather, they act as inert (nonmetabolizable) anions and, therefore, induce dilution acidosis in a manner analogous to that of isotonic saline. This whole problem is discussed in detail on page 44.

*Summary of the therapy of phase I*
The aim of phase I therapy is to expand blood volume and to prevent imminent shock or treat overt shock. The most readily accessible fluid for this purpose is either isotonic saline or an ECF replacement fluid, which should be started immediately in amounts of about 10 ml/kg during phase I (5 ml/kg/hr for 2 hr) in moderately dehydrated patients. In the severely dehydrated patient, approximately twice this amount is appropriate, but therapy in this case must be highly individualized depending on continuous monitoring of the circulatory variables. The intravenous route must always be used. The choice of fluids depends on the acid-base disturbance present in the patient and this can be deduced from the pathophysiology of the specific illness present. Patients with disorders known to produce metabolic alkalosis (e.g., pyloric stenosis) should receive isotonic saline, whereas those suspected of having either no acid-base disturbance or having metabolic

acidosis (e.g., diarrhea) should receive an ECF replacement fluid.

The end of the initial hydrating infusion marks the first formal feedback point (see Table 11), and in most patients a substantial improvement will be noted. In rare instances of severe dehydration, however, where the improvement is less than expected, blood transfusion or a plasma expander should be given at this point, the blood having been ordered for typing and cross matching at the time of admission (see the discussion in earlier paragraphs). If blood has not been ordered, it should be ordered promptly, and an additional 10 ml/kg of initial hydrating solution or 5 ml/kg of plasma expander should be continued. Some of these cases are likely to have severe hypotonic dehydration, and this should become evident as soon as the initial plasma sodium concentration value is reported from the laboratory. Were severe hyponatremia to be present (i.e., sodium less than 120 mEq/L) and the patient's circulatory status still only questionably adequate after the initial hydrating infusion, a hypertonic sodium solution should be considered in the subsequent therapy. This point will be discussed in conjunction with the therapy of phase II. The pathogenetic mechanisms underlying this particular therapeutic strategy have been discussed earlier.

In the uncomplicated dehydration patient, the time duration of phase I is 2 or more hours. No maintenance fluids are given during this time and certainly no potassium-containing fluids should be given until the initial plasma potassium concentration and the initial blood acid-base data are reported from the laboratory. This lapse will be corrected after the initial laboratory data are available, at which time the maintenance fluid required for the first hospital day will be given and the plan for phase II therapy will be made. The maintenance fluid aspect of this total therapeutic program can be computed according to the principles already outlined on page 68.

## THERAPY OF PHASE II—RESTORATION OF EXTRACELLULAR FLUID VOLUME

Once circulatory integrity is established, the next phase of therapy can be safely undertaken. This second phase is designed primarily to provide a substantial restoration of the depleted extracellular fluid and sodium stores as well as a partial, usually substantial correction of the abnormal plasma sodium concentration and the disordered acid-base status, assuming that the deviations of the initial sodium concentrations are not large. Special precautions are required for management for the hypernatremic patient, as will be spelled out later in the book.

## Theoretical considerations

As discussed previously, the ECF bears the major brunt of the total water deficit in all types of dehydration. In addition, when a significant potassium deficit is present, as is usually the case, the depletion of extracellular sodium stores comes about not only by a loss of sodium to the environment, but also by a further loss of sodium into the ICF in exchange for the potassium that has been lost to the environment. If all losses of sodium, potassium, and water could be safely replaced instantaneously, the organism would satisfactorily restore normal electrolyte composition and normal volumes of both the ECF and the ICF. But it is not safe to restore the large intracellular potassium deficits that are likely to be present as rapidly as the extracellular sodium and water deficits, since the large amounts of potassium that are required cannot be safely transported via the extracellular fluid in a short period of time without the risk of hyperkalemia.

The recognition of the need for *sequential* rather than *simultaneous* replacement of sodium and potassium deficits is fundamental to the formulation of specific recommendations for therapy of phase II and phase III. This point is illustrated with the aid of a specific example in Figure 33.

The figure shows two quantitatively different extremes of therapy that could be adopted for an isotonically dehydrated infant. Both sequences follow the general principle of rapid replacement of the sodium deficit and slower replacement of the potassium deficit. They differ in the amounts of sodium given. In sequence A, the entire water loss from the body is replaced in the *first step* (i.e., sum of phases I and II) as an isotonic sodium solution (either isotonic saline or an ECF replacement fluid). This procedure would restore extracellular fluid volume to normal and replenish completely the extracellular sodium stores, leaving the intracellular potassium deficit and the intracellular sodium excess as the remaining abnormalities.

In sequence B, the first step consists of replacement of only half the total extracellular fluid volume deficit by an isotonic sodium solution (this selection of half is arbitrary, but it has been chosen to illustrate the point). Following this, ECF volume and extracellular sodium stores would be increased but would still be less than

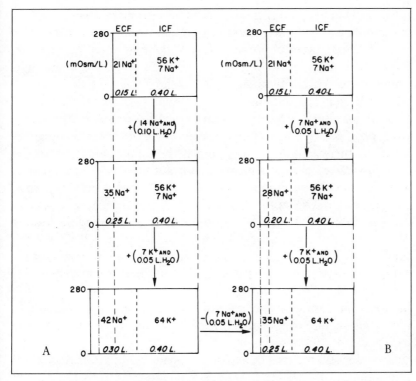

FIGURE 33. Quantitative consequences of sequential replacement of sodium and potassium deficits. The upper diagrams both represent an infant who has sustained an isotonic loss of 0.10 L/kg containing 7 mEq/kg each of $Na^+$ and $K^+$ (along with 14 mEq/kg of $Cl^-$ plus $HCO_3^-$). A. The first step (middle diagram) on the left shows the effects of the replacement of the *entire* ECF volume deficit in one step by an isotonic sodium infusion. ECF volume is thus restored to normal at 0.25 L/kg of body weight, and ECF sodium stores (previously 21 mEq/kg) are also normal at 35 mEq/kg. B. The first step (middle diagram) on the right shows the effects of replacement of only *half* of the ECF volume deficit with a commensurate amount of $Na^+$, so that ECF volume has risen to 0.20 L/kg and ECF sodium stores have risen to 28 mEq/kg. At the end of this step in each sequence, there is still 7 mEq/kg of sodium in the ICF, and the intracellular $K^+$ deficit remains. In the next step of each sequence (bottom diagram) the $K^+$ deficit is now restored with the "release" of $Na^+$ from the ICF, which reenters the ECF. On the right-hand sequence, the restitution of ICF $K^+$ deficits leads to a normal value for ECF $Na^+$ content (35 mEq/kg), and along with a retention of water from the intake (0.05 L/kg), the body fluids are completely restored to normal. In the second step (bottom diagram), in the left-hand sequence, the restitution of the $K^+$ deficit is accompanied by a similar ICF-to-ECF migration of sodium, which is retained along with a proportional amount of water from the intake, so ECF volume is now supernormal at 0.30 L/kg, and the ECF sodium is likewise supernormal at 42 mEq/kg. Subsequent renal excretion of this excess ECF water and sodium leads to a restitution of completely normal body fluids.

normal. There remains an extracellular volume and sodium deficit, and an intracellular potassium deficit and sodium excess.

In the second step in both sequences, potassium replacement (in phase III) is now provided. In sequence B, the uptake of potassium now releases intracellular sodium, which reenters the ECF, restoring completely the remaining extracellular sodium deficit. An additional amount of water is then retained from the exogenous intake (provided by the maintenance allotment of water being given simultaneously) by the kidney, and ECF volume now rises to the final normal value. In sequence B, intracellular potassium is also restored, and the sodium released by the cells also enters the extracellular fluid. At this point there is a supernormal value for extracellular sodium content. If this sodium were retained by the kidney along with an equivalent volume of water (again from exogenously administered sources), the patient would end up with a supernormal volume of extracellular fluid. There is convincing evidence indicating that transient retention of sodium and water does in fact occur during this phase of therapy in patients who are treated in this manner. Subsequently, normal renal control is regained, the excess extracellular sodium and water are excreted, and restoration of the volume and composition of the body fluids to normal takes place.

The preceding considerations are important in formulating quantitative recommendations for fluid therapy in phase II. Clearly, if the entire water deficit were repaired with a sodium-containing fluid, one would run the risk of edema incident to replacement of the potassium deficit during phase III, as is shown on sequence A of Figure 33. Alternatively, if one assumes that half of the cation loss is sodium and the other half is potassium, one can partially restore the sodium deficit and the accompanying extracellular water deficit rapidly, and then allow the remaining repair of the extracellular fluid to occur more slowly as the potassium deficits are repaired. In effect, this therapeutic approach envisions one rapid large step that partially expands extracellular fluid, followed by a series of smaller, slower steps that are intended to approach the normal value in a sort of asymptomatic fashion. The above course of action rests upon the fundamental assumption that the potassium deficit is of a magnitude equivalent to the sodium deficit, and that intracellular exchanges of the type illustrated in Figure 33 occur with potassium loss. Since one can never be sure in any given patient that the deficits of sodium and potassium are precisely or even approximately equal, it would seem most prudent to adopt some midcourse between the two extremes depicted in Figure 33—namely, to restore extracellular volume during phase II by, let us say, two thirds of the estimated deficit. The patient is then reevaluated at the end of the phase with respect to the adequacy of ECF expansion as well as the detection of the presence of any major degrees of potassium deficit.

The foregoing presents the theoretical underpinnings of this phase of therapy, while emphasizing that the best course of action is to minimize treatment on the basis of intelligent interpretation of feedback data, with reasonable therapy. Patients deserve this individualization of theory, and the foregoing is meant to point the way toward an individual blending of two potential tools (theoretical principles coupled with intelligent assessment of feedback data) to generate an individualized therapy for a given patient with a specific set of disorders.

## Specific formulations of therapy

Specific formulation of deficit therapy for phase II is primarily dependent on the type of dehydration present, as revealed by the interpretation of the initial plasma sodium concentration—isotonic, hypertonic, or hypotonic—and secondarily modified by the nature of the acid-base derangement, if any. Three therapeutic programs for phase II corresponding to the three major types of dehydration will be presented in the following paragraphs.

## Isotonic dehydration

In cases of isotonic dehydration, the aims of therapy of phase II can be realized by continuing the infusion of the initial hydrating mixture, albeit at a slower rate, so that by the end of phase II the patient will have received from one half to two thirds of the total estimated water loss as an isotonic sodium-containing fluid. For example, an infant with severe isotonic dehydration (e.g., about 15% of the initial body weight) has a total water deficit of 150 ml/kg. The initial hydrating infusion (20 ml/kg) has already been given over the first 2 hr of therapy. The aim of Phase II would be to continue the expansion of the ECF volume isotonically, so a total volume between 70 and 100 ml/kg is reached within 18 to 24 hr after admission to the hospital. Thus, the rate of initial hydrating infusion (isotonic saline or extracellular replacement fluid during phase I) would be slowed commensurately during phase II, so that at the end of phase II, the patient would have received the amounts of water and electrolyte shown in Table 13. Correspondingly smaller amounts would be given to infants with less severe degrees of dehydration in accordance with the initial estimates of the severity of dehydration.

The fluid program covers only the deficit portion of phase II. Maintenance fluids must be provided for the entire first day of treatment. In general, they may be provided as soon as circulatory integrity is assured. In the infant, normal maintenance therapy would consist of providing 100 ml of a maintenance fluid mixture for each 100 Cal expended. Since the estimated caloric expenditure of the (nonfebrile) infant is about 100 Cal/kg, the maintenance requirements per kilogram would be 100 ml of water, 2.5 mEq of sodium, 2.5 mEq of potassium, and 5 g of glucose (see p. 72). In general, in patients with acidosis or prerenal azotemia, it is unwise to administer any potassium until these abnormalities are largely corrected (see the discussion of precautions for potassium administration in the following paragraphs). Therefore, maintenance potassium is omitted or reduced according to biochemical monitoring during the first day of therapy, and normal maintenance requirements could be met by 100 ml/kg of a maintenance fluid containing sodium and chloride at 25 mEq/L in 5% dextrose (Table 5).

Finally, attention must be given to any *abnormal maintenance requirements* that occur during phase II—for example, owing to ongoing diarrhea, vomiting, intestinal suction losses, and other losses. Of course, the best course of action is to stop such losses, if possible. If an infant or child who is vomiting or having diarrhea is not fed by mouth, the abnormal loss will often cease entirely. Abnormal losses occurring during phase II should be replaced as outlined in Table 8. However, the potassium component of the abnormal maintenance requirements should be omitted for this period unless one is confident that the circulation is stable and that prerenal azotemia or metabolic acidosis are being corrected. A summary of the entire fluid program covering phase I and II encompassing the first hospital day for this particular patient is shown in Table 13.

### Hypotonic dehydration

If the initial plasma sodium concentration indicates a hypotonic (plasma sodium concentration less than 130 mEq/L) rather than isotonic dehydration, the therapy of phase II may be modified from that discussed in preceding paragraphs by providing an extra allowance for sodium. It is conceptually useful to divide the re-

TABLE 13. Fluid Therapy for an Infant with Severe Isotonic Dehydration

| Phase | Fluid Description | $H_2O$ (ml/kg) | $Na^+$ (mEq/kg) | $K^+$ (mEq/kg) | $Cl^-$ (mEq/kg) | $HCO_3^-$ (mEq/kg) | Dextrose (gm/kg) |
|---|---|---|---|---|---|---|---|
| Phase I (0–4 hr) | 20–30 ml/kg of extracellular replacement fluid* | 20–30 | 3.1–4.6 | 0 | 2.6–3.8 | 0.5–0.8 | 0 |
| Phase II (2–24 hr) | 80–100 ml/kg of extracellular replacement fluid* | 80–100 | 12.0–15.4 | 0 | 10.3–12.9 | 2.0–2.5 | 0 |
| | 100–125 ml of $Na^+$ maintenance fluid (without $K^+$)† | 100–125 | 2.4–3.0 | 0 | 2.4–3.0 | 0 | 5.0–6.3 |
| | Abnormal maintenance | | | As required | | | |
| Phase III (2–4 days) | 125–150 ml/kg/day of $Na^+$ + $K^+$ maintenance fluid,† plus 3 mEq KCl/kg/day (1.5 ml potassium chloride) | 125–150 | 3.0–3.6 | 6.0–6.6 | 9.0–10.2 | 0 | 6.3–7.5 |
| | Abnormal maintenance | | | As required | | | |

*Approximately two thirds and one third of the amounts shown would be appropriate for moderate and mild degrees of dehydration, respectively. Extracellular replacement fluid is used in cases with metabolic acidosis or those with no acid-base disturbance; isotonic saline is used in cases with metabolic alkalosis (see Table 12).
†See Table 5.

quirements for Phase II of therapy of hypotonic dehydration into two categories. One must first correct the existing hypotonic dehydration to an isotonic one, and, second, proceed to correct the now isotonic dehydration so as to achieve a final normal extracellular fluid volume and composition. In other words, one must calculate: (1) the amount of sodium required to convert the hypotonic dehydration to an isotonic dehydration, this amount of sodium to be given as a hypertonic solution, and (2) the amount of sodium and water required to expand the ECF isotonically.

The first component of the sodium requirement, the amount to correct the hypotonicity, can be readily computed according to the following general equation derived from osmometric principles:

$$(mEq/kg)\ Na^+\ required = (Normal\ plasma\ [Na^+]\ -\ observed\ plasma\ [Na^+]) \times TBW$$

In this equation, the normal plasma sodium is known and the observed plasma sodium concentration is measured at the time of admission to the hospital. (Since the initial hydrating infusion, which contains about 154 mEq/L, will likely raise the initial plasma sodium slightly, a value of 135 mEq/L may be used as the normal plasma sodium concentration, rather than the 140 mEq/L in the preceding equation to take account of this effect.) Total body water (TBW) is the remaining unknown in the above equation, and it must be estimated as usual from the clinical criteria. This can be done with reasonable accuracy, however, provided one recalls the expected normal values for total body water of the patient according to age (see Figure 1), and further, recognizes that the signs of dehydration are likely to be more marked in any given degree of total body water loss if the dehydration is hypotonic than if it is isotonic.

For example, an infant has signs indicating severe dehydration and an initial plasma sodium concentration of 115 mEq/L. The normal TBW estimated for such a patient would be about 0.65 L/kg. In view of the severe degree of dehydration and the severe degree of hypotonicity (113 mEq/L), a reasonable estimate of the water deficit would be about 10 percent of the body weight, rather than the 15 percent that would be the case if the infant had an isotonic dehydration of comparably severe proportions. Thus, the estimated TBW of the hypotonically dehydrated infant would be 0.65 L/kg − 0.10 L/kg = 0.55 L/kg. Using this equation, the mEq of sodium per kilogram of body weight required to restore the plasma sodium to normal without effecting any change in TBW could be computed as follows:

$$\begin{aligned}
\text{Amount of Na}^+ \text{ (mEq/kg)} &= (125 - 113 \text{ mEq/L}) \times 0.55 \text{ L/kg} \\
&= 22 \text{ mEq/L} \times 0.55 \text{ L/kg} \\
&= 12 \text{ mEq/kg}
\end{aligned}$$

Were this amount of sodium to be provided as *dry salt* (without water), the dehydration would be converted from a (severe) hypotonic to a (moderate) isotonic one, the plasma sodium concentration after the administration of the salt load rising to 135 mEq/L or so. It should be pointed out that in this process, the ECF volume would be expanded despite the absence of any exogenous water intake, since the rising osmolarity of the extracellular fluid would effect a water movement from the intracellular fluid into the extracellular fluid, contracting the former while expanding the latter (see Figure 5).

In practice, one can come close to this hypothetical dry salt administration by the use of hypertonic sodium solutions—for example, 5% sodium chloride (855 mEq/L each of $Na^+$ and $Cl^-$) or an additive sodium bicarbonate solution (1 mEq/L ml equivalent to 1000 mEq/L) or some mixture of these two. The volume of hypertonic sodium fluid required to restore the plasma sodium concentration to normal in hypotonic dehydration can be calculated by the following general expression:

$$\text{ml of fluid required per kg} = \frac{\text{mEq Na}^+ \text{ needed per kg}}{\text{mEq/ml of Na}^+ \text{ in the fluid to be used}}$$

It should be noted that the same argument (see p. 44) concerning the possible adverse effects of dilution acidosis on a preexisting metabolic acidosis is as valid in this case as in the case of isotonic dehydration. However, with hypertonic infusions the water that produces the dilution is derived not from the infusate itself but from the ICF incident to the osmotically induced transfer of non-bicarbonate-containing water from that compartment into the ECF. To avoid this problem, one should use a mixture of 5% sodium chloride and hypertonic (1 mEq/ml) sodium bicarbonate to provide three fourths of the sodium as chloride and one fourth as bicarbonate. The volumes of each of these fluids needed in the final mixture can be calculated from the preceding equation.

The equation illustrates how a severe hypotonic dehydration

can be converted to an isotonic dehydration. In practice, one may sometimes wish to go ahead and administer the hypertonic sodium infusion to effect this conversion as a single step. The practical decision to do so is based entirely on clinical factors, the most important of which is whether the severe hyponatremia is thought to be producing signs or symptoms that demand prompt relief. The rate of such an infusion is determined by the intensity of the signs and symptoms; in general, 4 to 8 hr seems reasonable.

Many physicians, particularly those who are inexperienced with the use of hypertonic sodium solutions, prefer a more leisurely correction using isotonic saline. But to repair a severe hyponatremia with isotonic saline seems to be overly cautious and physiologically cumbersome; to achieve correction in this way requires the kidney to conserve the salt and excrete the water—in other words to make "dry salt" from isotonic sodium solutions in amounts exactly equal to those calculated from the replacement equation. For example, in the example given, 25 mEq/kg of dry salt are required; this would be equivalent to about 250 ml/kg of isotonic saline, assuming a complete renal separation of retained sodium from the excreted water. Aside from this very large extra volume of fluid that would need to be infused, it may be asking too much of the kidney to perfectly separate and excrete the water, which is not needed, from all of the salt, which is needed.

A grossly inadequate response of the circulation to the therapy (isotonic sodium) in phase I in a subject whose admission data shows severe hyponatremia would be an important factor in deciding that a hypertonic sodium infusion should be given. If such were the case, the infusion should be given over a period of approximately 4 to 8 hr via the intravenous route. After completion of the infusion (i.e., within about an hour), the plasma sodium concentration should be measured again to ascertain whether the desired result has been produced. (The failure to achieve the plasma sodium concentration within a few mEq/L predicted from the preceding equation is evidence for ongoing sodium losses of major proportions—e.g., obligatory sodium loss via the urine as in adrenocortical insufficiency, and this possibility should be explored.)

Signs or symptoms suggesting overhydration of cells of the central nervous systems and, in particular, convulsions would be another indication for hypertonic sodium infusion. However, in contrast to the situation in acute water intoxication, in which neuronal cell volume increases very rapidly, convulsions and other signs of water intoxication are not often seen in uncomplicated hypotonic dehydration, probably because the time needed for hypotonicity to develop is much longer, and neuronal cell volume has probably become readjusted (see Figure 28).

Thus, whether one actually proceeds with the administration of the hypertonic solution is basically a clinical decision. The theory underlying the computation of the sodium deficit remains valid and can be incorporated into an alternative therapeutic program, as will be explained. Were the plasma sodium concentration to be restored to normal by an initial hypertonic infusion, the second component of phase II therapy for hypotonic dehydration would consist of an isotonic expansion of the still contracted extracellular fluid along the lines already outlined for the therapy of isotonic dehydration. Since the restoration of plasma sodium concentration to normal would have already produced some expansion of the ECF owing to osmotic transfer of water from the ICF, less exogenous isotonic sodium-containing fluid would be required for this step than for an isotonic dehydration in which the TBW loss was comparable.

In most instances of hypotonic dehydration, the hypertonic sodium infusion is not given separately first, followed by the isotonic infusion. Rather, both components are in effect given together by computing the requirements separately and mixing the two replacement fluids together in a single bottle. Let us again consider the infant discussed earlier on page 124 who has signs of severe hypotonic dehydration and metabolic acidosis. Therapy for phase I, consisting of 20 ml/kg of ECF replacement fluid, has been given over a period of 2 hr. The two components of the sodium requirement for phase II are then calculated from the measured plasma sodium concentration (113 mEq/L) and the estimated TBW of 0.55 L/kg. The *first component*—that required to restore the plasma sodium concentration to normal—is computed from the equation (see page 124) and is 12 mEq/kg. This should be given as a mixture of 9 mEq of hypertonic NaCl and 3 mEq of $NaHCO_3$. The second component of the sodium requirement is 40 to 60 ml/kg of ECF replacement fluid; when added to the amount of solution already administered in phase I, this fluid would provide sufficient sodium and water to effect a significant isotonic expansion to a value approximating the desired level at the end of phase II. Thus, rather than administering a hypertonic fluid first, followed by the isotonic fluid later, the two fluids could be mixed together and the mixture administered over the time course of phase II to simultaneously correct the plasma sodium to normal and expand the ECF volume by the requisite amount. Table 14 gives a treatment program for severe hypotonic dehydration in an infant.

It is obvious that the amount of sodium needed to repair hypotonic dehydration is large whether the procedure is carried out in a sequence or in combination, and if administered rapidly, might constitute a potential threat to the heart. This risk might be particularly relevant to a very rapid infusion of a hypertonic solution alone and seems more likely in the adult than in the infant. Indeed it is my belief that in severe hypotonic dehydration the risks attributed to profound circulatory collapse, if real, are sufficient to override the hypothetical risk of circulatory overload from the infusion, assuring no intrinsic cardiac disease.

In addition to the deficit therapy, normal and abnormal maintenance requirements must also be met for the first day of treatment. Requirements for each of these are formulated following the general principles previously discussed (see page 68) and illustrated in the preceding discussion of isotonic dehydration.

### Feedback information in isotonic or hypotonic dehydration

The end of phase II marks the second formal point for the clinical and chemical reevaluation of the patient. Clinically, the signs of dehydration should be receding and the patient should look better. This is usually most apparent in the filling out of the face and the brightening of the eyes. Skin turgor should be improved, and mucous membranes should be less dry. An accurate body weight at this point is essential to judge the degree of expansion of the extracellular fluid and should reveal a value of 5 to 20 percent over that on admission. Circulatory signs and urine flow should have stabilized during phase II.

One of the first patients with dehydration whom the author managed as a green intern was an infant with moderately severe diarrheal disease. In taking the history, the mother, a poorly educated but very astute observer, remarked that the baby "didn't look right out of his eyes." After 24 hr of fluid therapy, the child had improved greatly, and the mother noted that he now "looked normal out of his eyes." Over the author's subsequent 3 decades of experience, this glazed appearance of the eyes of dehydrated infants, which is assumed to represent an increased concentration of protein due to diminished water content of the tears or other eye fluids, has proved to be a very valuable sign; its disappearance

TABLE 14. Fluid Therapy for an Infant with Severe Hypotonic[a] Dehydration

| Phase | Fluid Description | H$_2$O (ml/kg) | Na$^+$ (mEq/kg) | K$^+$ (mEq/kg) | Cl$^+$ (mEq/kg) | HCO$_3^-$ (mEq/kg) | Dextrose (gm/kg) |
|---|---|---|---|---|---|---|---|
| Phase I (0–4 hr) | 20–30 ml/kg of extracellular replacement fluid[b] | 20–30 | 3.1–4.6 | 0 | 2.6–3.8 | 0.5–0.8 | 0 |
| Phase II (2–24 hr) | 40–60 ml/kg of extracellular replacement fluid[b] to which are added 10 ml sodium chloride 5%[c] and 3 ml/kg sodium bicarbonate[c] | 53–73 | 18.1–21.2 | 0 | 14.2–16.8 | 4.0–4.4 | 0 |
| | 100–125 ml/kg Na$^+$ + K$^+$ maintenance fluid (without K$^+$)[d] | 100–125 | 2.4–3.0 | 0 | 2.4–3.0 | 0 | 4.0–6.3 |
| | Abnormal maintenance | | | As required | | | |
| Phase III (2–4 days) | 125–150 ml/kg of Na$^+$ + K$^+$ maintenance fluid,[d] plus 1.5 ml/kg potassium chloride (3 mEq/kg/day) | 125–150 | 3.0–3.6 | 6.0–6.6 | 9.0–10.2 | 0 | 6.3–7.5 |
| | Abnormal maintenance | | | As required | | | |

[a]Plasma [Na$^+$] = 113 mEq/L.
[b]Approximately two thirds and one third of the amounts shown would be appropriate for moderate and mild degrees of dehydration, respectively. Extracellular replacement fluid is used in cases with metabolic acidosis or those with no acid-base disturbance; isotonic saline is used in cases with metabolic alkalosis (see Table 12).
[c]Calculated by the method explained in the text; in metabolic alkalosis, all sodium for correction of hyponatremia would be given as chloride.
[d]See Table 5.

corresponds well with successful therapy. Indeed, this is an example of one of those seemingly masterful tricks of the great old clinicians, who as if by telepathic knowledge, can pronounce that a previously dehydrated infant is obviously improved simply by looking at the infant through the doorway from the hall.

Chemically, plasma sodium concentration should be within or very close to the normal range. The blood urea nitrogen and plasma creatinine concentrations show substantial falls if prerenal azotemia is present initially. Acid-base status should likewise show substantial improvement, but in moderate or severe initial disorders, it will likely not be completely restored to normal by the end of phase II. Thus, in patients with metabolic acidosis, the plasma $PCO_2$ will likely still be low, although blood pH may actually be nearly or completely normal at this point. This is due to the delayed readjustment of the normal respiratory control and is the rule rather than the exception during recovery from metabolic acidosis. Indeed, if the plasma bicarbonate concentration, initially low, were completely normal at the end of 24 hr, the blood pH would very likely be alkaline owing to the lag in respiratory readjustment with its attendant low $PCO_2$. With the moderate amounts of bicarbonate therapy recommended, this trend toward alkalemia is avoided or minimized since the expectation is that the plasma bicarbonate concentration will not be fully restored by the end of phase II. Specific acid-base therapy will be discussed later in the book.

In patients with metabolic alkalosis, there should likewise be a substantial improvement in acid-base status at the end of phase II in that the initially high bicarbonate levels should show an appreciable and significant fall. It is, however, unlikely that a completely normal value has been achieved at this point, since complete recovery from metabolic alkalosis, even if the originating factor can be controlled, generally takes several days under optimal conditions. Blood pH will be alkaline at the end of phase II, although less so than the value obtained on admission.

Plasma potassium concentration, if initially high-normal or frankly elevated, as is likely in dehydration associated with prerenal azotemia and metabolic acidosis, will have fallen to low-normal or perhaps even frankly low values signifying the need to begin replacement of body potassium deficits (phase III). In initially alkalotic patients, plasma potassium may be low on admission and fall even further during phase II—a point that will be discussed further below.

*Hypertonic dehydration*

Hypertonic dehydration in infants poses one of the more complex electrolyte problems the pediatrician is called on to manage. This is because of the frequency of neurologic abnormalities, including convulsions, that occur in infants with hypertonic dehydration, especially when the chemical abnormalities are rapidly corrected. The origin of these neurologic abnormalities is not known with certainty. Minute multiple hemorrhages in the brain substance probably contribute to them. Physiologically, most attention has been focused on the seizures during treatment. They have been likened to water intoxication, though in that instance the osmolarity of the body fluids is rapidly lowered from normal to subnormal values, whereas in the therapy of hypertonic dehydration it is lowered from supernormal to normal values. A possible clue to the origin of the neurologic findings observed during rapid recovery from hypertonic dehydration may lie in the osmotic behavior of the erythrocyte. It has been pointed out earlier (see Figure 28) that erythrocytes abruptly exposed to a hypertonic environment shrink, but with time they seem to reestablish a normal cell volume. When such an adapted cell is suddenly exposed to a normal osmotic environment, it swells to supernormal proportions, and only later is cell volume readjusted to normal. If neurons show a behavior similar to that of erythrocytes, one might invoke an abrupt increase in cell volume to supernormal size as the immediate cause of neurologic signs when hypernatremia is abruptly corrected. Such a hypothesis, although unproven, is attractive in bearing out the analogy with acute water intoxication.

Regardless of the mechanism, it is a common clinical impression that convulsions attending recovery from hypertonic dehydration in infants may be diminished although not necessarily completely avoided, if the initially high values for the extracellular osmolality and plasma sodium are more gradually rather than abruptly readjusted to normal. To manipulate the plasma sodium concentration with respect to the magnitude as well as the rate of change in such a patient requires considerable attention to the details of the fluid therapy coupled with good laboratory feedback. In general, it seems that the safest course is to try to reduce the plasma sodium concentration by no more than 10 mEq/L per day during therapy. Thus, if the initial plasma sodium concentration were 170 mEq/L, a total of 3 days would be required to achieve a stepwise fall to the normal value of 140 mEq/L.

Such relatively slow correction is usually possible (primarily) because most infants with hypertonic dehydration do not show marked contraction of the extracellular fluid. This is because the deficits of sodium are relatively well maintained owing to the rising osmolarity of the body fluids, which causes the ICF to share to a significant degree in the total water deficit (see Figure 26). This explains why the hypertonically dehydrated infant is rarely in overt shock and often does not show many of the signs of dehydration to any significant degree despite the fact that the loss of body water may have been substantial. This deceptive nature of dehydration follows from the fact that most of the signs of dehydration are related more closely to the volume deficit of the extracellular fluid than they are to the volume deficit of the total body water.

Specific therapy for phase I (i.e., specifically aimed at bolstering the circulation) may or may not be required for such infants on admission to the hospital depending on the clinical assessment of the patient. However, if the circulatory status is completely adequate, an intravenous infusion of an ECF replacement solution should be started and continued at a slow rate pending the results of the laboratory data. If there is any doubt about the status of the circulation and if the signs of dehydration are present to a moderate degree, some rapid restoration of the ECF volume is likely to be desirable, and this should consist of the ECF replacement fluid. This choice is dictated by the fact that diarrheal dehydration with attendant metabolic acidosis is by far the most common cause of hypertonic dehydration in pediatrics. It should be noted that an infusion of say 20 ml/kg of this or any other isotonic fluid prior to obtaining a laboratory value later that reveals a high plasma sodium concentration (at the end of phase I) will not produce any significant decrease in the initially high value for the plasma sodium concentration. Thus, for example, in the average moderately dehydrated infant with a plasma sodium of 170 mEq/L, the infusion of 20 ml/kg of an isotonic sodium solution would dilute the initially high plasma sodium value by no more than 2 to 3 mEq/L.

To achieve a slow correction of the abnormal plasma sodium concentration, therapy of phase II must be considerably modified from that of isotonic or hypotonic dehydration, with respect to the time course of administration and the types of solution used.

The practice noted earlier in managing fluid therapy of the LBW infant by merely stating a concentration of a solution and an adequate description of the treatment given is also prevalent in the treatment of hypernatremia. This practice is exemplified by such statements as, "the patient was treated with quarter-normal saline" (or some other solution identified only by its concentration of sodium). Such a statement is obviously incomplete since one wishes to know not only the concentration of sodium but also the volume of the solution so infused. The total amount of water and the total amount of sodium are the only physiologically relevant variables.

Restoration of plasma sodium concentration from high to normal values requires that a hypotonic fluid be used; but some sodium should be present in the fluid, since despite the hypernatremia, the patient with this disorder usually has a decreased body content of sodium. In many cases, a fluid containing sodium in a concentration of 25 to 35 mEq/L (in 5% dextrose) is quite useful—that is, a fluid similar to that used for maintenance purposes but lacking potassium. In general, such a fluid provided in the amounts of 60 to 70 ml/kg/day over a period of several days will provide adequate sodium for replacement of sodium deficits and will produce the desired degree of gradual fall in plasma sodium concentration (Table 15). Depending on the degree of acidosis present, the sodium in this fluid can be given with varying mixtures of chloride and bicarbonate. Certain commercially available fluids that may be used for the preceding purposes are discussed later (see p. 150).

During the period of correction of the high plasma sodium concentration, maintenance fluids must also be provided. However, the usual practice of providing 200 ml of maintenance fluid per 100 Cal expended requires modification. This modification is necessary, because the kidney of the hypertonically dehydrated patient is under a strong stimulus from *antidiuretic hormone* (ADH) secretion due to the hypertonic ECF, and, therefore, the urine volume is obligatorily small. Under normal conditions, the customary maintenance water allotment is 55 ml of water per 100 Cal for urine volume. Because of the strong antidiuretic hormone stimulus due to the hypertonic body fluids, this allowance for urine volume is unquestionably excessive. The result is that if the usual allowance is given, the dilution of the plasma sodium concentration will occur much more rapidly than is desirable.

Suppose, for example, that the obligatory urine volume of such a patient is 30 ml/100 Cal, rather than the usual 55 ml/100 Cal. If 55 ml/100 Cal were given, a net retention of "pure water" of about 25 ml/100 Cal would occur. This is approximately one third of the total volume of water being given for the repair of deficits. The result is therefore a much more rapid dilution of the plasma sodium concentration than is anticipated. In the author's opinion, this is the single most common error in the formulation of the fluid therapy for the patient with hypertonic dehydration. In general, maintenance water requirements for patients with hypertonic dehydration should be reduced to about two thirds to three fourths of the usual amount—that is, 65 to 75 ml/100 Cal, rather than the usual 100 ml/100 Cal (see Table 15).

It is usually not necessary to administer potassium during the first several days of therapy when the primary aim is to correct the plasma sodium concentration. Indeed, since patients with hypertonic dehydration do not generally develop large potassium deficits (see Table 9), relatively small amounts of potassium may be needed for replacement of deficits.

Further, the plasma potassium concentration is usually normal or even elevated, particularly when the degree of acidosis is significant. In general, it is best to omit or reduce the potassium intake during the period of correction of the plasma sodium and to rely on subsequent potassium therapy, which the patient with hypertonic dehydration usually needs, in phase III.

Finally, any abnormal maintenance requirements (e.g., ongoing diarrhea) should be met; such replacement should follow the principles already outlined (see p. 75). Here again, it is essential that the amount of replacement fluid given be accurately estimated, since water from any source may lead to overly rapid dilution by virtue of the loss of renal flexibility incident to the hypernatremia. In general, it is unnecessary to replace the potassium abnormally lost unless the plasma potassium concentration falls below the normal values.

*Feedback in hypertonic dehydration*
Feedback information in the management of phase II of hypertonic dehydration should consist of serial daily measurement of the plasma electrolytes and acid-base status. A fall in the plasma sodium occurring at the rate more or less predicted (10 mEq/L/day) signifies that the overall therapeutic program is adequate. It is often useful to monitor the urine volume, and if necessary, to adjust the maintenance requirements to take account of the actual urine volume of the patient under these conditions. The body weight should slowly increase, and the blood urea nitrogen and plasma creatinine concentrations, if initially elevated, should fall as the ECF volume is corrected.

Serial clinical observation of the patient is essential. Infants with

TABLE 15. Fluid Therapy for an Infant with Severe Hypertonic[a] Dehydration

| Phase | Fluid Description | $H_2O$ (ml/kg) | $Na^+$ (mEq/kg) | $K^+$ (mEq/kg) | $Cl^-$ (mEq/kg) | $HCO_3^-$ (mEq/kg) | Dextrose (gm/kg) |
|---|---|---|---|---|---|---|---|
| Phase I (0–2 hr) | 20 ml/kg of extracellular replacement fluid[b] | 20 | 3.1 | 0 | 2.6 | 0.5 | 0 |
| Phase II (2 hr–4 days)[c] | 60–75 ml/kg/day of $Na^+$ maintenance fluid (without $K^+$)[c] or 60–75 ml/kg/day of Dextrose 5% in water plus 24 ml of sodium bicarbonate | 60–75 | 1.4–1.8 | 0 | 1.4–1.8 | 1.4–1.8 | 3.0–3.8 |
| | 75 ml/kg/day of $Na^+$ or $Na^+$ + $K^+$ maintenance fluid[d] | 75 | 1.9 | (1.9) | 1.9(38) | 0 | 3.8 |
| | Abnormal maintenance | | | As required | | | |
| Phase III (4–6 days)[e] | 125–150 ml/kg/day of $Na^+$ + $K^+$ maintenance fluid,[d] plus 1 ml/kg of potassium chloride (2 mEq/kg/day) | 125–150 | 3.0–3.6 | 5.0–5.6 | 8.0–9.2 | | 6.3–7.5 |
| | Abnormal maintenance | | | As required | | | |

[a] Plasma $[Na^+]$ = 170 mEq/L.
[b] May not be required when admission findings do not suggest marked contraction of plasma volume.
[c] Duration of phase II varies with degree of hypernatremia present initially; in general, a fall of plasma $[Na^+]$ of 10 mEq/L/day is desirable.
[d] See Table 5.
[e] Phase III follows completion of phase II and provides usual maintenance requirements in addition to an extra provision of $K^+$ to repair deficits.

hypertonic dehydration are often lethargic and may be comatose. The deep tendon reflexes may be exaggerated. Tremors are frequent, and convulsions and tetany-like seizures may appear if the sodium concentration is readjusted too rapidly. But even when the plasma sodium concentration is being slowly returned to normal, these disturbing central nervous system signs may appear. In some instances, definite hypocalcemia is found; it should be treated by the addition of 10 to 20 ml of 10% calcium gluconate to the daily infusion. The seizures may be severe enough to warrant anticonvulsive medication, in which case diazepam is a useful drug.

## SOME PRINCIPLES OF THE TREATMENT OF ACID-BASE DISORDERS
### General principles
Thus far, the therapy of acid-base disorders has received little specific attention, aside from the general recommendation of using a fluid containing either bicarbonate or a bicarbonate-precursor for phases I and II in patients with acidosis; a sodium chloride solution should be used similarly in dehydrated alkalotic patients.

In most instances of metabolic acidosis and alkalosis, this approach is quite satisfactory, although there are occasional instances in which the intensity of the acid-base disorder seems to call for a more aggressive attack. The reader is reminded here that there are several general principles that apply to the management of all acid-base disorders. These principles may be summarized under the following heads.

1. *Identify and control cause.* If possible, identify and control the underlying cause of the specific acid-base disorder. One example of this would be the use of an appropriate insulin regimen in diabetic ketoacidosis; with the restoration of normal carbohydrate metabolism, the ketone body anions ($\beta$-hydroxybutyrate and acetoacetate) will no longer be generated, and those remaining in the body fluids will be metabolized. The metabolism of these anions, like other oxidizable organic anions (lactate, gluconate, acetate, and so forth) leads to the endogenous generation of bicarbonate. For this reason, these organic anions have been referred to as "potential" bicarbonate; in those instances in which it is possible to reestablish normal metabolism by some specific therapeutic maneuver, such as insulin in diabetic acidosis or restoration of an inadequate circulation in lactic acid acidosis owing to shock, the respective

organic anions will be transformed via metabolism from "potential" bicarbonate to "actual" bicarbonate.

A number of other examples could be cited in which the primary acid-base disturbance, whether metabolic or respiratory, can be controlled by specific therapy against the causative disorder. In respiratory disorders, the primary therapy must always be targeted toward normalizing the disturbed alveolar ventilation—for example, institution of artificial ventilation in respiratory acidosis.

In diabetic ketoacidosis as well as in lactic acid acidosis due to hypoperfusion, appropriate therapy directed at the primary factor (e.g., insulin and expansion of blood volume, respectively) should, theoretically, correct the acidosis entirely—that is, in the complete absence of any renal function—since the metabolic transformation of the respective organic anions would be replaced mol for mol by bicarbonate. In terms of formal conceptualization, it is useful to classify all varieties of metabolic acidosis into those in which the *only* mechanism for correction (this term being used here as previously defined on p. 36) is via the regeneration of body bicarbonate stores through acidification of the urine, and those in which correction can be achieved completely via the metabolism of organic anions to bicarbonate, the metabolism, hence, occurring entirely by *extrarenal* means (exemplified by diabetic ketoacidosis or lactic acidosis).

2. *Improve compensatory mechanisms.* Attempt to improve upon the efficacy of the compensatory mechanisms if they are believed to be impaired, and in addition, ensure that the corrective mechanisms are operating to their maximal ability. In a patient with metabolic acidosis and relatively poor respiratory compensation, for example, improving the corrective mechanisms would restore the diminished renal perfusion incident to concomitant dehydration through a vigorous rehydration. It is well recognized that the kidney of a dehydrated salt-depleted patient is limited in its ability to acidify the urine and, hence, to correct metabolic acidosis. In metabolic alkalosis, on the other hand, the renal limitation on bicarbonate excretion imposed by hypochloremia calls for the provision of adequate amounts of chloride as well as cations to promote the excretion of bicarbonate. In passing, it should be noted that those limitations on bicarbonate excretion in metabolic alkalosis due to cation deficiency may be present in respiratory alkalosis and, if so, re-

quire the same considerations with respect to provision of an adequate cation supply.

### Specific therapy of acidotic states

It is only after the preceding general approaches have been implemented, where feasible, that one should consider a specific direct attack on the abnormal blood pH by the use of exogenous acid or base. Two fundamental questions must be answered in order to formulate a physiologically appropriate program. Although the present state of knowledge is far from sufficient to allow completely satisfactory answers to these questions, the topic deserves brief discussion because of its fundamental importance. The questions are

1. How serious should the distortion in blood pH be in order to justify specific therapeutic intervention through the administration of large amounts of exogenous acid or base?
2. How much exogenous acid or base should be given and over what period of time should it be administered?

With respect to the first question, it should be obvious at the outset that on a priori biologic grounds, there can be no specific, single value for an abnormal blood pH beyond which one would institute specific therapy, although there is an understandably widespread yearning among clinicians for biology to be so simple. However, the lack of a simple answer to this complex question has not prevented various authorities to promulgate rules for instituting specific therapeutic regimens based on specific alterations of blood pH. The problem arises most frequently in the treatment of acidotic syndromes in the newborn infant. Specific values for blood pH below which specific therapy is instituted seem to vary from pH 7.20 down to 7.00, depending on the particular authority consulted. Although such rules are simplistic, they are genuine attempts to assist the front-line clinicians who must face the problem that severe acidemia is associated with fatal outcome. Even though this association may not represent a direct cause-and-effect relationship, the prudent clinician is unlikely to want to test this hypothesis in the severely acidotic patient. See Author's Notes 3, page 162.

It is neither fair nor sufficient to dismiss such an important question with trivial answers, even, as in the present case, when no substantive answers are available. With this particular question, it seems to the author that the so-called experts in acid-base physiology ought to listen more closely to the clinical authorities since the latter at least have the benefit of a very large clinical experience. In following such advice, it is important, however, to recognize that when these highly experienced physicians decide to administer large doses of bicarbonate in acidosis, they do so not only on the basis of a specific abnormal laboratory value, but, consciously or not, they are also taking account of a whole constellation of clinical signs and symptoms presented by the patient and are evaluating these against their own long experience. Thus, the answer to the first question is not a single numerical value for blood pH, it is a complex clinical assessment that often happens to correlate roughly with a numerical value for blood pH that is of the order of 7.20 or below.

### The bicarbonate replacement equation

Accepting the premise that specific treatment is indicated in life-threatening acidemia, we move to the second question—how much and how fast should one try to correct the abnormality? This is a two-part question, neither of which can be answered easily or simply. An oft quoted formula for the computation of the amount of bicarbonate needed for correction takes the following general form:

$$\text{Amount of } HCO_3^- = ([\text{Met Comp}]_f - [\text{Met Comp}]_i) \times f \times BWt$$

where $[\text{Met Comp}]_f$ and $[\text{Met Comp}]_i$ are the final and initial concentrations of plasma bicarbonate concentration (or whole blood base excess) and $f \times BWt$ is some assumed constant value of the body weight, often equated with one of the major subdivisions of the body water.

This equation closely resembles the replacement equation used to compute the amount of sodium given as a hypertonic solution to correct hyponatremia:

$$\text{Amount of } Na^+ = ([Na]_f - [Na]_i) \times f \times BWt$$

In the author's opinion, the superficial similarity of these two equations has conferred a physiologic dignity on the bicarbonate equation that it emphatically does not deserve. Indeed, a comparison of the sodium replacement equation and the bicarbonate replacement equation is very instructive in revealing the fallacies of the latter.

The sodium replacement equation has been tested extensively

and found to be valid, and the term $f \times BWt$ conforms very closely to the total body water.

This does not mean that the volume distribution of sodium is the TBW. Indeed, if one were to inject a tracer amount of isotopic sodium, its acute volume distribution would more likely approximate the ECF. The reason $f \times BWt$ equals TBW in the sodium replacement equation is that sodium and its accompanying anions account for nearly all of the effective osmolarity of the ECF (see p. 9); hence, $2 \times [Na^+]$ is an excellent approximation of $[Osm]$. The sodium equation is really a derivative of the osmotic replacement equation: Amount of Osm $= ([Osm]_f - [Osm]_i) \times f \times BWt$, where $[Osm]$ refers to the concentration of nonpenetrating solutes. Since $[Osm] = 2 \times [Na^+]$, the above equation, divided by 2 on either side, yields the sodium equation. The factor $f \times BWt$ in the sodium equation is sometimes called the *osmotic distribution of sodium* to differentiate it from its true *volume distribution*, which, as in the isotopic experiment quoted, would be close to the ECF.

The assumptions underlying the validity of the sodium replacement equation in correcting hyponatremia (or the converse equation for water replacement in the correction of hypernatremia), are (1) sodium is metabolically inert, and once it is infused, it can be neither created nor destroyed; and (2) the patient has no ongoing losses of sodium during the infusion. Of course, the amount of sodium so computed must be given as a strongly hypertonic solution, usually at a 3 or even a 5 percent concentration so as not to significantly affect the value for TBW.

The bicarbonate equation has very different attributes. First, bicarbonate can be both created and destroyed in the body. It is created whenever $H^+$ is lost to the environment, as in the production of gastric acid or in the acidification of the urine. It is also created if there is a significant degree of ongoing metabolism of organic ions, such as lactate, acetate, gluconate, and so forth. Finally, bicarbonate can be created by certain buffer reactions (see Tables 2 and 3).

On the other hand, there are situations in which bicarbonate is either lost or consumed. The most obvious losses occur when there is a loss of small-intestinal juices or when an alkaline urine is passed. It can also be consumed in the course of buffering (see Table 2) of the usual normal production of metabolic acid, a situation that may be greatly exaggerated in certain disease states, most notably diabetes, and so forth, in which organic acids are produced in large amounts.

Thus, unlike sodium, bicarbonate is capable of either net production or net destruction (or loss). In metabolic acidosis, in which a patient is likely to receive an infusion of bicarbonate, it is probable that bicarbonate is being lost continuously by buffer reactions due to an exaggeration of ongoing acid production or loss of bicarbonate. In a patient with respiratory acidosis, it is most probable that bicarbonate is being produced as a result of buffer reactions incident to a rapidly rising plasma $PCO_2$.

The next objection to the bicarbonate equation concerns the value to be assigned to the term $f \times BWt$. In reviewing the accumulated experience with this problem, it is impressive to note that the published values for $f$ are generally not only highly variable in any one study but are also from study to study. Thus, the published range of values varies from about 25 percent to values as high as 70 percent of the body weight—that is, approaching or even exceeding the probable TBW. Although the causes of these discrepancies are only partly understood, it is noteworthy that the highest values for $f$ were reported in cholera patients, where ongoing stool losses of bicarbonate are notoriously large. But a more subtle process may also be at work as well in that bicarbonate replacement must regenerate both bicarbonate and nonbicarbonate buffers of the blood, of the ISF (which has little nonbicarbonate buffer), and of the ICF (which has an abundance of nonbicarbonate buffer). Some recent studies suggest that the behavior of the nonbicarbonate buffers of the ICF is not a linear function of the change in the ECF buffers. If this is so, any single linear equation for replacement of bicarbonate in all compartments will simply not work. Finally, one should note that an appreciable but variable fraction of any dose of infused bicarbonate is almost immediately lost by buffering through interaction with the blood nonbicarbonate buffers:

$$HCO_3^- + HBuf \longrightarrow Buf^- + H_2CO_3 \longrightarrow CO_2 + H_2O$$

When one considers all these factors, it is hardly surprising that the bicarbonate equation fails more often than it succeeds. Furthermore, it is poor pedagogy to perpetuate this mathematical disguise of our physiologic ignorance.

It is all well and good to discard one approach, but it is incumbent on those who do so to substitute a better one. To this end, the author feels that given the present state of knowledge of bicarbonate dynamics in the body fluids, one should adopt a strictly empirical approach to the problem of bicarbonate replacement by giving a reasonable amount over a reasonable time period, assessing the result, and, on the basis of that experience, develop a reasonable subsequent dose for the next time period. This process should be repeated until the judgment is made that no further exogenous bicarbonate is needed.

In metabolic acidosis, a reasonable initial amount would be 2 to 4 mEq/kg, depending on the severity of the acidemia over a period of 4 hr. This amount may be added directly to an ongoing infusion estimated to be given over the following 4 to 6 hr. (In no case can the rapid injection of a bolus of bicarbonate be condoned, at least in this general clinical setting.) At that point, blood acid-base feedback information should be obtained and the next dose—a larger or smaller dose, or perhaps even none—should be administered over a similar time period. The same approach applies to treatment of respiratory acidosis.

In both instances, one must guard against an overly rapid correction of plasma bicarbonate concentration. In metabolic acidosis, it is well recognized that respiratory compensation, once established, does not abruptly cease when blood pH reaches normal. Rather, there is almost always a transient period of about 12 hr during which plasma $PCO_2$ returns progressively to normal. If the plasma bicarbonate concentration is abruptly restored to normal while the plasma $PCO_2$ is still low, an alkalemia, which could be quite severe, would result. In respiratory acidosis, on the other hand, effective ventilatory assistance may well cause the plasma $PCO_2$ to fall abruptly, and with an increasing plasma bicarbonate concentration, alkalemia would ensue. As is discussed in the following paragraphs, an abruptly induced alkalemia is not a benign event; rather, it may set the stage for serious neuromuscular or cardiac abnormalities.

Conceptually, the distinction should be made between those varieties of metabolic acidosis in which there is an accumulation of organic anions that under proper conditions can be metabolized to bicarbonate and those in which the cause of the acidosis is fundamentally owing to a loss of bicarbonate (or a gain of HCl). These two varieties can be distinguished from each other on etiologic grounds and can be confirmed by an examination of the plasma anion pattern. Thus, in the first group, plasma UA is elevated, usually almost reciprocally with the degree of fall in plasma bicarbonate concentration; in the second group, plasma chloride concentration rises reciprocally without the fall in plasma bicarbonate concentration. This distinction is important in formulating bicarbonate therapy, since in the first group of disorders there is often a reasonable expectation that the normal metabolic pathway can be re-established (e.g., by giving insulin in uncontrolled diabetes) and, if it is, the organic anions will be metabolized, and an equivalent amount of bicarbonate will be generated. Hence, exogenous bicarbonate therapy in this group in which return to normal metabolism can be anticipated should be viewed as a temporary measure to tide the patient over a severe acidemia until the other measures take effect. In such cases, if one were to give enough exogenous bicarbonate to fully correct the plasma bicarbonate concentration to normal and to fully restore metabolism at the same time, the end result would be a supernormal bicarbonate concentration. Given the prevailing low plasma $PCO_2$ (see the discussion in earlier paragraphs), these maneuvers would unquestionably produce a severe degree of alkalemia.

### Specific treatment of alkalotic states

Thus far, only bicarbonate replacement in acidotic states has been discussed. It is useful to consider the subject of specific treatment of respiratory and, especially, metabolic alkalosis, since these topics generally receive relatively scant attention, whereas there is a wealth of information and opinion about the treatment of acidotic states.

Respiratory alkalosis rarely needs specific treatment; the exception is in the acute variety in which there is a rapid onset of hyperventilation producing an abrupt fall in plasma $PCO_2$ and an accompanying rise in blood pH. Most commonly this occurs as an emotional response (such as to the sight of blood) or in response to a low $PO_2$ at high altitude. In susceptible individuals, it may be accompanied by an increased neuromuscular excitability, evident by a positive Chvostek's or Trousseau's sign, and an increased predisposition to seizures or paresthesias. In highly susceptible individuals, syncope may result. In such instances of the so-called hyperventilation syndrome, rebreathing of expired $CO_2$ by using a small paper bag is an effective way of managing the problem.

Acute symptomatic respiratory alkalosis occurs in some individuals who fly abruptly from sea level to a high altitude. Dizziness, light headedness, and similar complaints are frequent. Renal compensation takes several days, and certain individuals may be quite uncomfortable until blood pH falls toward or to normal. After one such personal experience, the author tried to acclimatize himself at sea level by a 3-day course of acetazolamide prior to departure on a subsequent trip. This produced a mild fall in plasma bicarbonate concentration; when hyperventilation occurred owing to the low $PO_2$ at altitude, the degree of alkaline shift of blood pH would be expected to be considerably less and symptoms of acute hyperventilation thereby avoided. Although none of the symptoms attributed to alkaline pH appeared, a troublesome and very persistent paresthesia of the foot (a well known side effect of acetazolamide) makes it doubtful that this bit of physiologic manipulation will be tried again.

The specific treatment of metabolic alkalosis by the direct infusion of an acidogenic substance has not received the attention that it deserves. In recent years, this particular acid-base disorder, occurring alone or as a part of a mixed disorder, has emerged fairly frequently and often to a severe degree, especially in complex postoperative cardiac patients. In many of these patients, it is often impossible to identify a primary single etiology, but such factors as prior large bicarbonate infusions, large and repeated doses of ethacrynic acid or furosemide, and large mobilizations of edema (leading to contraction alkalosis) are the most likely culprits. In older patients, a syndrome of multiple organ failure involving heart, lung, liver, and kidney, occurring in such a rapid, predictable fashion as to be thought of almost as a domino effect, is a well recognized entity in many surgical intensive care units. A related syndrome accompanied by metabolic alkalosis is also not uncommon in chronically ill, postoperative cardiac infants.

Traditional teaching holds that the kidney will correct metabolic alkalosis, given enough cation and, especially, enough chloride, but under the simplest of conditions, such as gastric alkalosis, these measures require about 3 to 6 days to fully correct the abnormality. If one has this much time to allow the kidney to correct the disorder, one should allow it to do so. But in more complex postoperative patients with metabolic alkalosis associated with multiple organ failure, the need for further surgical intervention may arise rather suddenly. Under such conditions, the possibility of imposing a transient hyperventilation during the induction of general anesthesia on an already elevated plasma bicarbonate concentration would lead to a severe, abrupt further rise in blood pH. In this setting, the incidence of severe cardiac arrhythmias will markedly increase.

It would be desirable to obtain at least a partial correction of the alkalosis prior to subjecting such patient to general anesthesia, but to do so would require the infusion of an acid or a substance that will generate an acid after its metabolism. Parenteral ammonium chloride preparations are still available but are rarely used, although in the absence of liver disease (such as in infants with pyloric stenosis and gastric alkalosis), up to 6 mM/kg/day have been given without clinically adverse effects. Arginine hydrochloride is a very attractive alternative acidogenic substance, because the arginine is metabolized to urea, generating hydrochloric acid in the process. At present, a commercial preparation of arginine hydrochloride is not available. However, most endocrinologists have arranged for the availability of a sterile intravenous preparation of arginine hydrochloride for growth hormone studies. Large hospital pharmacies with appropriate facilities can readily manufacture this type of preparation.

As in the case of bicarbonate, the matter of dosage is an empiric one. There is no single theory supported by good evidence that permits one to compute dosage from purely theoretical principles. Lacking this, the author continues to favor the empirical approach by recommending a reasonable quantity of arginine: HCl—(2 to 4 mEq/kg) to be given over a 4 to 6 hr period—added to the ongoing infusion, assessing the effects of this maneuver on the acid-base status at the completion of the infusion, and using this information as a guide for further therapy. Since the experience with such acidifying agents is far less than with alkalinizing agents, it seems prudent to monitor the patient very closely and to institute such treatment only when a more leisurely pace seems an undesirable choice, owing to a pressing need to intervene with some other procedure potentially likely to affect adversely the already complex abnormalities of the acid-base status of the patient.

## THERAPY OF PHASE III—RESTORATION OF BODY POTASSIUM DEFICITS

Body potassium deficits are sustained almost entirely at the expense of the ICF since over 98 percent of the total body potassium resides in that compartment. Yet the ECF is the only route by which potassium can be resupplied to cells, and its concentration of potassium is normally very low compared with that of the ICF. Therefore, in the repair of potassium deficits one must take account of the fact that relatively large amounts of this ion must be provided to the cells through the vehicle of the ECF without producing a serious or even a transient increase in the concentration of potassium in the ECF.

## Precautions in potassium administration

The oral route is preferable for potassium replacement, since its use tends to minimize the risks of hyperkalemia during repair. However, when oral intake is contraindicated, because of vomiting, diarrhea, intestinal obstruction and so forth, the parenteral route must be used. Thus, at least during the initial part of phase III, the parenteral route must be relied upon principally or completely. Parenteral potassium administration always involves some risk of hyperkalemia, but this can be minimized if certain precautions are observed. First, it is unwise to administer potassium unless the general circulatory status, and, in particular, the renal circulatory status, is adequate and stable, since the normal kidney provides a safety valve for the excretion of potassium if the plasma potassium concentration becomes elevated. Second, parenteral (or oral) potassium replacement is contraindicated when the plasma potassium concentration is already elevated; replacement should be undertaken cautiously if at all when a serious degree of acidosis is present. The latter precaution arises from the fact that the acidosis itself tends to cause the plasma potassium concentration to rise, and in an unstable therapeutic situation, it is always possible for the acidosis to become worse. This is not to say that when feedback information at the end of phase II shows there has been substantial improvement in the correction of acidosis, that potassium replacement cannot begin; rather, it is to caution against overzealous or premature replacement of potassium deficits in situations in which the chances of hyperkalemia are increased. Third, although body potassium deficits may be large, approaching the deficits of sodium, one cannot safely replace them as rapidly as one replaces sodium deficits. Thus, a patient may have a body potassium deficit of the order of 10 mEq/kg (see Table 9). To attempt a total replacement of this deficit in a single 24-hr period is not only unwise but it may be inefficient as well, since the kidney is likely to excrete much of the potassium presented in an amount as large as this.

For all of the reasons given, no more than about 3 mEq/kg/day should be used for replacement of potassium deficits unless there are unusual or extenuating circumstances (such as obligatory large losses of potassium in the urine). Thus, the average time for replacement of potassium deficits is about 3 to 4 days with 3 mEq/

kg/day of potassium over and above any normal or abnormal maintenance requirements being given continuously over each of these days. A final precaution concerns the concentration of potassium in the infusate, which should not exceed 40 to 50 mEq/L, except in extraordinary circumstances. This is more a practical than a theoretical point, and it derives from the fact that a transient increase in drip rate, if undetected, could suddenly flood the extracellular fluid with potassium if the concentration of potassium in the infusate were very high. This type of transient hyperkalemia, due to abrupt unpredictable changes in the rate of flow of the infusate (which may occur particularly in infants), can be minimized by keeping potassium concentrations in the infusate at levels lower than about 50 mEq/L.

*Specific formulations of therapy*

Therapy in phase III, the duration of which may be 3 or more days, should consist of 3 mEq/kg of potassium as potassium chloride, together with an extra increment of water sufficient to provide for further expansion of the extracellular fluid, which is incident to the displacement of intracellular sodium as intracellular potassium is reaccumulated (see p. 118). Usually, these two requirements can be met by augmenting the usual daily maintenance fluid intake by 25 percent and adding 3 mEq/kg of KCl. This mixture, which now provides maintenance water and electrolyte requirements as well as potassium replacement and an additional increment of water for extracellular water expansion, should be given continuously intravenously throughout the entire 24-hr period for which it is intended. In addition, any abnormal maintenance requirements should also be met, following the general principles already outlined. In these cases, the replacement fluid may also contain potassium as well as other electrolytes and water in amounts sufficient to meet the ongoing losses.

In uncomplicated cases, the parenteral intake of potassium can be decreased as the oral intake of fluid is increased. Potassium chloride may be added to oral fluids in multiple small, divided amounts throughout the entire 24-hr period. If potassium-rich fluids are being ingested, no supplements may be necessary. In any event, one should consult dietary tables to ascertain the approximate level of potassium in the particular fluid being taken by the patient, and it should be supplemented, if necessary, so that the potassium intake of 3 mEq/kg/day for deficit repair plus the maintenance potassium requirements are being met by some combination of oral fluids or parenteral fluids. Very high concentrations of potassium in oral fluids should be avoided (i.e., more than 70 to 80 mEq/L, final concentration), since these produce pylorospasm and may induce vomiting.

Feedback information during and at the end of phase III should include daily weight of the patient and, periodically, chemical status of the plasma. Acid-base status should be completely restored by the end of phase III, and the plasma potassium as well as the plasma sodium and chloride concentrations and BUN and plasma creatinine concentration should be within the normal range.

### THERAPY OF PHASE IV—REPAIR OF NUTRITIONAL DEFICITS

The final deficits to be repaired are those incurred as the result of a period of suboptimal caloric intake and lack of exogenous protein intake. Once the patient is eating a full diet, the deficits of body fat and protein will be restored. Complications arise only when full oral caloric and protein intake cannot be taken—for example, in recurrence of moderate to severe diarrhea on refeeding of the patient. If the patient was previously well nourished, another period of exclusive parenteral therapy should be tried and the oral intake restarted more slowly, perhaps with a different feeding mixture. But not infrequently, such patients are already seriously malnourished or become so as multiple cycles of refeeding followed by recurrence of diarrhea continue. Under these conditions, the lack of a full caloric and protein intake becomes a serious, even life-threatening problem. In such patients, one may have to resort to the parenteral route as the main if not the sole route for the provision of calories and nitrogen as well as water and electrolytes. This technique is discussed in a subsequent chapter.

### COMMENTS ON THE MIXING OF INTRAVENOUS SOLUTIONS

#### Tailor-made solutions

The present-day clinician is faced with an array of commercially available intravenous fluids that are widely used in the management of the patient with dehydration in restoring the deficits of water, electrolytes, and so forth, as well as for the provision of maintenance requirements. Indeed, over the past several decades, there has been a marked change in practice in favor of using these commercially available premixed solutions; using the older method, a patient's requirements were estimated and a fluid tailor-made from a few widely available solutions and additives to meet those requirements.

There were some obvious advantages to this now largely discarded approach, the most notable being that the physician was forced to think in a more fundamental and appropriate physiologic mode than is now the case when premixed solutions are used. The system of fluid replacement using tailor-made solutions forced one to think of requirements as so many ml of water per kilogram, so many milliequivalents of electrolyte per kilogram, and so many calories per kilogram. A fluid containing the requisite amounts would be mixed from a few standard solutions (e.g., isotonic saline, glucose solutions, potassium and bicarbonate additives, and, occasionally, hypertonic saline). At one time, this practice was widespread, with the actual mixing being performed at the bedside; only casual attention was given to sterile technique and none to the addition of particulate matter, such as tiny bits of rubber that enter the solution when a needle is passed through a rubber stopper. By current standards, which call for mixing to be carried out in laminar flow hoods and in-line filters to remove particulate matter, this older practice was indeed primitive. The remarkable fact is that it seemed to be relatively safe; only rarely were cases encountered in which a contaminated bottle of mixed fluid was identified as the culprit in a septic patient. Nor were any clinically evident complications due to the infusion of particulate matter ever recognized (nor, for that matter, are they recognized even now as clinically significant). The reason for the relative rarity of septic complications was that the solution was mixed and given promptly, so that any bacteria it may have contained never achieved the logarithmic phase of their growth cycle. Any infused particulate matter is efficiently removed by the lung, which as we now recognize, has a great capacity for filtering blood-borne exogenous or endogenous particles (e.g., small emboli).

The real hazard in the do-it-yourself school of fluid mixing was the chance for human error that would lead to a major complication, such as inadvertent failure to add solute to a solution, thereby provoking a major hemolytic reaction. This safety problem plus the admitted convenience of having a sterile, quality controlled commercial line of intravenous solutions led to their nearly universal acceptance. In those hospitals having effective additive programs manned by trained pharmacists, one can still obtain tailor-made, expertly compounded solutions, although at greater expense. Because each patient's problems should be analyzed and treated individually, the author still recommends the individualized approach.

*Problems in the use of commercial solutions*

The current widespread use of commercial solutions, however, has created its own problems, and they are largely in the area of pedagogy. Specifically, prior to the introduction of the popular multiple-electrolyte solutions, one was likely to approach a given patient's needs by estimating the needs as $x$ ml/kg of water and $y$ mEq/kg of each electrolyte. Now we are likely to hear that the treatment of the patient consisted of "quarter-normal saline," of some commercial solution with a nondescript name, such as "omega solution." Such sloppy use of the language reflects a sloppy intellectual approach to the problem. The essential information in conveying information about treatment is the same now as it has always been—$x$ ml/kg of water and $y$ mEq/kg of each electrolyte given, and the period of time over which this has occurred; that is, we need to know the *volume* as well as the precise *composition* of each specific solution given as well as the duration of the infusion.

Regrettably, the manufacturers of the presently available commercial solutions have not made it easy to know or even to guess at the composition of most of the solutions that are available from the names they have bestowed upon them. In part, this is related to the purely business aspects of this highly competitive field; a strong trend in the development of these solutions over the years has been to take a basically simple solution containing, let us say, the amounts of sodium, chloride, and a bicarbonate-precursor approximating those of plasma and to add physiolocically insignificant amounts of potassium, calcium, and magnesium, thus creating a multiple electrolyte-containing solution. Each pharmaceutical company has spawned at least one family of such multiple electrolyte solutions, each bearing a family name followed generally by either an initial or a number. The specific names given to the various families of solutions are interesting, representing what must be the creative pinnacles of the marketing divisions of the various companies.

Invariably, the family name of each solution family consists of a prefix, *iso-*, *iono-*, *poly-*, or *plasma-*, and a suffix, *-sol*, *-sal*, *-lyte*, or *-ionic*. To differentiate one individual member of the family from another, the family name is often followed by an initial (e.g., *R* for replacement, *M* for maintenance) or by a number that most likely represents the concentration of total cations or some other constituent, although which one is not always apparent.

Table 16 gives some of the features of the commercial solutions by listing the compositions of those most widely used. They all contain the total cations at a final concentration approximating that of normal plasma, and they are therefore useful for replacement purposes. Maintenance solutions are discussed in the following paragraphs.

### Bicarbonate-precursors versus bicarbonate

The "window dressing" effect achieved by the addition of tiny amounts of potassium, calcium, and magnesium to create the isotonic polyelectrolyte solutions should not obscure the fact that these solutions differ from each other fundamentally only as to the details of anion composition. For example, in one—isotonic saline (so-called normal saline)—the anion is entirely chloride, whereas in others, one fifth to one third of the total anions is composed of one or more metabolizable organic anions (lactate, gluconate, acetate, or combinations of these). It is assumed that all of these anions represent potential sources of bicarbonate, since bicarbonate is an end product of overall metabolism in each case. However, to achieve this metabolic transformation, the following conditions must be fulfilled: (1) the various anions must be transported to the sites of metabolism (usually, but not exclusively, in the liver); (2) the particular metabolic pathway must not only be intact, but it must be capable of operating at the rates required for prompt conversion to bicarbonate; and (3) there must be no renal loss of the anion. This last point is almost never discussed; rather, it is universally assumed that there is 100 percent conversion of each of these precursors to bicarbonate, an assumption that has not been well documented in every case. Indeed, in the case of lactate, and probably the other organic anions as well, the renal threshold is rather low, and a significant loss into the urine is therefore likely.

Given all these premises concerning the use of metabolizable organic anions as bicarbonate sources, one might well ask why there is no large-volume commercial solution that contains bicarbonate itself. Indeed, the simplest approach to the disorders for which the fluids in Table 16 are made is to use a simple solution containing sodium at a normal plasma concentration with the anions distributed approximately as 25% bicarbonate and 75% chloride. This straightforward approach would eliminate the win-

TABLE 16. Multiple Electrolyte Solutions for Replacement (mEq/L)

| Solution | Na⁺ | K⁺ | Ca⁺⁺ | Mg⁺⁺ | NH₄⁺ | Cl⁻ | HPO₄⁼ | HCO₃⁻ = Precursor | Comment |
|---|---|---|---|---|---|---|---|---|---|
| 0.9% Sodium chloride solution | 154 | | | | | 154 | | | Abbott |
| 0.9% NaCl with variable KCl | 154 | 10, 20 30, 40 | | | | 74, 84, 94, 104 | | | Travenol |
| M/6 Na lactate solution | 167 | | | | | | | Lactate 167 | Cutter |
| Lactated Ringer's solution[a] (Hartmann's solution) | 130 | 4 | 3 | 3 | | 109 | | Lactate 29 | Various companies |
| Acetated Ringer's solution | 130 | 4 | 3 | | | 109 | | Acetate 108 | Various companies |
| Ringer's solution[a] | 147 | 4 | 4 | | | 156 | | | Various companies |
| Normosol-R[a] | 140 | 5 | 98 | 3 | | | | Gluconate 23 Acetate 27 | Abbott |
| Normosol-R pH 7.4 | 140 | 5 | 98 | 3 | | | | Gluconate 23 Acetate 42 | Abbott |
| Normosol-R/K[b] | 140 | 30 | 98 | 3 | | | | Gluconate 23 Acetate 42 | Abbott |
| Plasma-Lyte[a,b] | 140 | 10 | 5 | 3 | | 103 | | Lactate 8 Acetate 47 | Travenol |

| | | | | | | | |
|---|---|---|---|---|---|---|---|
| Plasma-Lyte 148[a] | 140 | 5 | | 3 | 98 | Gluconate 23 Acetate 27 | Travenol |
| Plasma-Lyte pH 7.4 | 140 | 5 | | 3 | 98 | Gluconate 23 Acetate 27 | Travenol |
| Isolyte E[a] | 140 | 10 | 5 | 3 | 103 | Acetate 49 Citrate 8 | American McGaw |
| Isolyte S[a] | 140 | 5 | | 3 | 98 | Acetate 27 Gluconate 27 | American McGaw |
| Isolyte S pH 7.4 | 141 | 5 | | 3 | 98 | Acetate 27 Gluconate 23 | American McGaw |
| Polyionic-R 148[a] (replacement solution) | 140 | 5 | | 3 | 98 | Acetate 27 Gluconate 23 | Cutter |
| Polyionic-R 148 pH 7.4 (replacement solution) | 140 | 5 | | 3 | 98 | Acetate 27 Gluconate 23 | Cutter |
| Polysal balanced electrolyte solution | 140 | 10 | 5 | 3 | 103 | Acetate 55 Gluconate 23 | Cutter |

[a] With or without 5% dextrose.
[b] With 5% dextrose.

dow dressing—the inclusion of tiny amounts of magnesium, calcium, and potassium in the commercial polyelectrolytes solutions—and would seem to be a sensible solution for initial rehydration of an isotonically dehydrated acidotic patient (see p. 115). Indeed, for many years the author has recommended the mixture of this solution for such patients, and, for want of a better name, called it "artificial extracellular solution."

Some years ago at the author's suggestion, the Abbott Laboratories manufactured and marketed an artificial extracellular fluid (Pediasol). This solution had the approximate electrolyte composition discussed in the text. It was directed (mistakenly in the author's opinion) exclusively to the pediatric patient, being put up only in 250-ml bottles. It proved to be a commercial failure for a variety of reasons. Such a solution, however, can be readily mixed as needed, preferably in a pharmacy equipped for sterile additive procedures. To mix one liter of such a solution requires 844 ml of isotonic saline, 24 ml of a $NaHCO_3$ additive (1 mEq/ml), and 5% dextrose, sufficient to make a final volume of one liter. The electrolyte composition of this fluid is 154 mEq/L of sodium, 130 mEq/L of chloride, and 24 mEq/L of bicarbonate.

When transferred to the commercial arena, this seemingly sensible approach fails on one very important criterion—cost. All the solutions shown in Table 16 are packaged in relatively inexpensive glass bottles and have a long shelf life. However, bicarbonate-containing solutions require a much higher quality of glass to achieve a comparable shelf life and to avoid leaching of impurities in the glass. Hence, the cost of a large volume parenteral solution containing bicarbonate makes it noncompetitive.

### Maintenance solutions and additives

So far we have been discussing only the sodium-rich replacement fluids. There are two other groups of commercial fluids which deserve consideration: (1) those that are useful for normal and abnormal maintenance purposes, and (2) the small volume additives.

A summary of the premixed, commercially available solutions that would meet or approximately meet normal maintenance needs is shown in Table 17. In general, these contain somewhat more sodium than potassium, but provided the various precautions discussed earlier with respect to maintenance therapy are observed, they are satisfactory. A second group of maintenance fluids having distinctly higher sodium than potassium concentrations is also available (Table 18). These were developed for patients with abnormal maintenance requirements, more specifically those with gastrointestinal losses, although the recommended approach spelled out earlier for these patients—that is, actually measuring the volume and the concentration of electrolytes in such losses and mixing a solution to meet them—is preferred. Lacking these measurements, one might find an appropriate commercial solution worthy of trial, provided there is careful monitoring to determine its efficacy.

A group of solutions that are useful alone or fortified with potassium are the fractional concentrations of isotonic saline (so-called half normal saline quarter normal saline, and so forth). If they are fortified with potassium in the amounts discussed earlier with respect to maintenance (see p. 75), such solutions are useful in meeting various normal and abnormal maintenance needs.

There are a great many additives available, containing varying concentrations of potassium, bicarbonate, sodium, and so forth (Table 19). Of these, only a few of the simplest ones are needed—that is, $NaHCO_3$ and KCl. A source of hypertonic NaCl, 3% or 5%, is also occasionally required for treating hypotonic dehydration. Finally, there is an occasional need for a phosphate additive for hypophosphatemia, and this is available as potassium phosphate additive.

Phosphate additives present a problem in the understanding of dimensions used to designate amounts of phosphate. Unlike all other ions we have been dealing with in intravenous solutions, the charge on the phosphate anion varies between $-1$ and $-3$, depending on the pH. Over much of the *physiologic* pH range, the valence varies between $-1$ and $-2$ (i.e., $H_2PO_4^-$ and $HPO_4^=$), as is summarized by the following equation:

$$PO_4^\equiv \rightleftharpoons \underbrace{HPO_4^= \rightleftharpoons H_2PO_4^-}_{} \rightleftharpoons H_3PO_4$$

*Physiologic pH Range*

Over the physiologic range of pH, the following equation for the two forms of phosphate anion may be written as follows:

$$pH = 6.8 + \log \frac{HPO_4^=}{H_2PO_4^-}$$

Table 17. Multiple Electrolyte Solutions for Normal Maintenance Purposes (mEq/L)

| Solution | Na$^+$ | K$^+$ | Ca$^{++}$ | Mg$^{++}$ | NH$_4^+$ | Cl$^-$ | HPO$_4$ = | HCO$_3^-$ Precursor | Comment |
|---|---|---|---|---|---|---|---|---|---|
| 0.2% NaCl with 5% dextrose and variable K$^+$ | 34 | 0, 10, 20, 30 40 | | | | 34, 44, 54, 64, 74 | | | Various companies |
| 0.33% NaCl plus 0.15% KCl in 5% dextrose | 56 | 20 | | | | 76 | | | Various companies |
| Ordway's solution: 0.2% KCl, 0.15% NaCl in 3.5% dextrose (also called pediatric electrolyte solution) | 26 | 27 | | | | 53 | | | Cutter |
| Plasma-Lyte M[b] | 40 | 16 | 5 | 3 | | 40 | | Acetate 12 Lactate 12 | Travenol |
| Plasma-Lyte 56 | 40 | 13 | | 3 | | 40 | | Acetate 16 | Travenol |
| Plasma-Lyte 56 in 5% glucose | 40 | 13 | | 3 | | 40 | | Acetate 16 | Travenol |
| Electrolyte #48[c,d,e] (pediatric maintenance solution) | 25 | 20 | | 3 | | 24 | 3 | Lactate 23 | Various companies |

| Solution | | | | | | | Anion | Company |
|---|---|---|---|---|---|---|---|---|
| Electrolyte #75[b,c] (also called maintenance solution) | 40 | 35 | | | 48 | 15 | Lactate 20 | Various companies |
| Electrolyte #2[c,d] | 56 | 25 | | 6 | 56 | 12.5 | Lactate 25 | Travenol |
| Electrolyte #4[e] | 30 | 15 | | | 23 | 3 | Lactate 20 | Travenol |
| Normosol-M[b] | 40 | 13 | 40 | 3 | | | Acetate 16 | Abbott |
| Ionosol-B[b,d] | 57 | 25 | 49 | 5 | | 13 | Lactate 25 | Abbott |
| Polyonic M 56[a] (maintenance solution) | 40 | 13 | | 3 | 40 | | Acetate 16 | Cutter |
| Polysol M (maintenance solution) | 40 | 16 | 5 | 3 | 40 | | Acetate 12 / Lactate 12 | Cutter |
| Electrolyte #2 (Butler's formula)[b,d] | 55 | 23 | | 5 | 45 | 13 | Lactate 31 | Cutter |
| Isolyte-H[b] | 40 | 13 | | 3 | 43 | | Acetate 16 | American McGaw |
| Isolyte-M[b] | 40 | 35 | | | 40 | 15 | Acetate 20 | American McGaw |
| Isolyte-P[b] | 25 | 20 | 3 | | 23 | 3 | Acetate 23 | American McGaw |
| Isolyte-R[b] | 40 | 16 | 5 | 3 | 41 | | Acetate 24 | American McGaw |

[a] With or without 5% dextrose.
[b] With 5% dextrose.
[c] With 10% dextrose.
[d] With 10% invert sugar.
[e] With 5% invert sugar.

TABLE 18. Multiple Electrolyte Solutions for Abnormal Maintenance Purposes (mEq/L)

| Solution | $Na^+$ | $K^+$ | $Ca^{++}$ | $Mg^{++}$ | $NH_4^+$ | $Cl^-$ | $HPO_4^=$ | $HCO_3^-$ Precursor | Comment |
|---|---|---|---|---|---|---|---|---|---|
| 2 1/1 Dextrose and half-strength lactated Ringer's solution | 65 | 2 | 1 | | | 54 | | Lactate 14 | Various companies |
| 2½% dextrose and half-strength Ringer's solution | 74 | 2 | 2 | | | 78 | | | Various companies |
| 0.45% NaCl | 77 | | | | | 77 | | | Various companies |
| 3% KCl and 4.5% NaCl[d] | 77 | 40 | | | | 117 | | | Travenol |
| 0.45% NaCl with variable K+ in 5% dextrose | 77 | 0, 10 20, 30 40 | | | | 77, 87 97, 107 117 | | | Various companies |
| Electrolyte #1[d,e] | 79.5 | 36 | 4.5 | | | 63 | | Lactate 60 | Travenol |
| Electrolyte #3[d] | 62.5 | 17.5 | | | 70 | 150 | | | Travenol |
| Ionosol-D/Cm[a] (duodenal) | 138 | 12 | 5 | 3 | | 108 | | Lactate 50 | Abbott |
| Ionosol-G+ (electrolyte #3)[d] | 63 | 17 | | | 70 | 151 | | | Various companies |
| Ionosol-D+[d] | 80 | 36 | 5 | 3 | | 64 | | Lactate 60 | Abbott |
| Electrolyte #1 (modified duodenum solution) | 80 | 36 | 5 | 3 | 63 | | | Lactate 60 | Cutter |
| Isolyte-G[b,c] | 65 | 17 | | | 70 | 150 | | | American McGaw |
| Multiple electrolyte | | | | | | | | | |
| #1[d] | 80 | 36 | 5 | 3 | | 64 | | Lactate 60 | American McGaw |
| #2[c] | 58 | 25 | 6 | | | 51 | 13 | Lactate 25 | American McGaw |

[a]With or without 5% dextrose; [b]With 5% dextrose; [c]With 10% dextrose; [d]With 10% invert sugar; [e]With 5% invert sugar.

TABLE 19. Summary of Additives and Miscellaneous Solutions

Sodium salts
  Sodium chloride (2.5 or 4.0 mEq/ml)
  Sodium chloride 3% (513) mEq/L)
  Sodium chloride 5% (855 mEq/L)
  Sodium acetate (2.0 or 3.0 mEq/ml)
  Sodium lactate (4.0 or 5.0 mEq/ml)
  Sodium bicarbonate (1.0 mEq/ml)
  Sodium bicarbonate 7.5% (44.6 mEq/50 ml)
  Sodium bicarbonate 5% (595 mEq/L)
Potassium salts
  Potassium chloride (1.5, 2.0, 2.5 or 3.0 mEq/ml)
  Potassium acetate (2.0 or 3.0 mEq/ml)
  Potassium phosphate (3 mM/ml)
Calcium salts
  Calcium chloride (10%)
  Calcium gluconate (10%)
  Calcium gluceptate (4.5 mEq $Ca^{++}$/5 ml)
Other
  Magnesium sulfate (50%)
  Ammonium chloride (3.0 or 4.0 mEq/ml)

Consider first a solution with a pH of 6.8. Under these conditions, the equation would be

$$6.8 = 6.8 + \log\frac{HPO_4^{2-}}{H_2PO_4^-} = 6.8 + \log\frac{1}{1} = 6.8 + 0 = 6.8$$

In other words, at pH 6.8, phosphate exists in equimolar amounts of $HPO_4^=$ and as $H_2PO_4^-$. Recalling the relationship between a milliequivalent and a millimol, a solution at pH 6.8 containing 1 mM of each form of phosphate would contain 2 mEq of $HPO_4^=$ and 1 mEq $H_2PO_4^-$.

This situation may be compared to that of a phosphate solution at pH 7.4 in which the equation would be

$$pH = 6.8 + \log\frac{HPO_4^=}{H_2PO_4^-}$$

$$7.4 = 6.8 + \log\frac{HPO_4^=}{H_2PO_4^-}$$

or

$$\log\frac{HPO_4^{2-}}{H_2PO_4^-} = 7.4 - 6.8 = 0.6$$

Solution of this equation by taking the antilogs of both sides shows that at pH 7.4, there is 4 mM of $HPO_4^=$ for every millimol of $H_2PO_4^-$. Thus at this pH, the $HPO_4^=$ would contribute 8 mEq (4 mM $\times$ 2 mEq) per liter, while the $H_2PO_4^-$ would contribute 1 mEq (1 mM $\times$ 1 mEq) per liter. Put another way, at pH 7.4, 5 mM/L of phosphate would exert a total negative charge of 9 mEq. Thus, if 5 mM of phosphate at pH 7.4 is equivalent to 9 mEq, 1 mM would have an average equivalence of 9 $\div$ 5 or 1.8 mEq per millimol. If one knows the number of millimols of phosphate at pH 7.4, the number of milliequivalents contributed by phosphate can be readily computed by multiplying by 1.8.

The point of the preceding discussion is to illustrate that the valence of phosphate is pH dependent, and for that reason one cannot specify a given number of millequivalents of phosphate anion without also specifying the pH. The appropriate procedure for considering phosphate requirements or when ordering phosphate replacement is to do so exclusively in terms of millimols and not in terms of milliequivalents. If the millimols required are specified, it is easy to compute the volume of a given additive needed to supply it. But if a given number of milliequivalents is specified without simultaneously specifying pH, it is meaningless. Even if pH is specified, the arithmetic to translate the requirement to millimols tends to become confusing and unnecessary.

AUTHOR'S NOTES

1. The otherwise healthy LBW or VLBW infant presents a striking example of the concept of "homeostasis through growth" when one considers renal solute excretion. Owing to their rapid rate of growth, there is a quantitatively larger diversion of substances (such as potassium, phosphate, protein, and to a lesser degree, sodium and chloride) derived from a full enteral intake into the synthesis of new body tissue than in older infants. Thus, on a formula delivering 200 Cal/day and a *potential* solute load of 40 mOsm/day, a 1500 g infant will reduce the *actual* solute excretion by 1 mOsm/g of weight gain or about 20 mOsm/20 g weight gain per day. If the same infant were fed the same formula under conditions where growth did not occur, the total solute load, comprising predominantly urea and electrolytes, would all become available for excretion. Thus, growth diverts half the total load, owing to the deposition of new tissue, and this markedly influences the magnitude of renal excretion of solutes directly and the renal excretion of water indirectly.

The rapid rate of growth in these infants also provides the only practical setting in which the water requirements for growth assumes any quantitative importance. In the preceding example, a 20 g daily weight gain would likely be associated with the daily deposition of 12 to 15 ml of water, depending on the proportions of fat (which is anhydrous) and lean body mass (which is about 80% water) being laid down. However, the rate of metabolism under these conditions is also high, so the water generated by the oxidation of foodstuff approximates the water being deposited in the newly formed tissue, and, hence, this fraction cancels out the water requirement for growth.

2. Students often seem to have the impression that fluid therapy for a given patient, at least for the first three phases, can be worked on admission by resorting to complex equations, tables, and other reference data. They seem to think that once this master plan is generated, it is to be followed to the letter by administration of the various prescribed fluids to the patient, and all will be well. It is easy to understand how this attitude is acquired, since the texts in the field, including the present one, necessarily try to dissect the physiologic complexities in order to present them in some reasonably clear and understandable way. Generalizations are inevitable. What is missing is the emphasis on modification, often significant modification, of the initial plan for an individual patient in accord with what will be referred to here as feedback data. Put another way, the author believes that the student should be given some physiologically sound methods by which a given phase of fluid therapy can be generated. This initial plan is the one that is the most sensible with respect to the physiologic facts at hand, but it is important to recognize that this plan also rests on some major assumptions and is therefore not to be treated as holy writ. Once a given plan is put into operation, the

systematic accumulation of feedback information may well point to a significant modification of the original plan; if this is the case, the appropriate modification should by all means be made. Furthermore, successive revisions must be made according to continuing assessment of feedback information until an ultimately satisfactory plan is achieved. In other words, what may appear to the student to be a rigorous exercise in clinical science is in fact a series of partly scientific and partly empirical steps that the physician takes, based on his best clinical and physiologic judgment coupled with intelligent collection and interpretation of feedback data.

3. Some years ago, the author had the occasion to participate in a panel discussion composed of a group of internationally recognized authorities on acid-base physiology. One of the questions presented to the panel was "what specific biochemical or clinical abnormalities could be expected from a low pH"? The panel hemmed and hawed, and reasoning from the well-known fact that since the extracellular and, probably, the intracellular pH values are very closely regulated in health, concluded that considerable degrees of physiologic disorder ought to be expected if pH deviated from the narrow range of normal. Finally, however, one of the more prescient members of the panel cut through all of these non-answers with the refreshing admission that no one really knew the answer to the question being posed, and that so far as he was concerned, a very acid blood pH simply turned protoplasm to Jell-O®!

# 5. *Parenteral Nutrition in the Pediatric Patient*

The provision of all nutrients in amounts sufficient to promote overtly normal growth in infants is a relatively recent innovation in the field of fluid therapy. Because of its importance, this subject deserves treatment in any book on fluid therapy.

Although parenteral nutrition has been the subject of great interest to pediatricians for many years, the practical feasibility of delivering a complete or nearly complete diet with each constituent present in its most elementary chemical form was nearly impossible using peripheral veins. Only with the seminal work of Dr. Stanley J. Dudrick, who perfected a method for the safe insertion and long-term maintenance of central venous catheters, has effective parenteral nutrition become possible. Such a route of delivery effectively solved the problem inherent in the composition of the dietary infusate—that it had an osmolarity about six times that of plasma, owing largely to the great amounts of glucose needed to meet the caloric requirement in a reasonable volume of fluid. Whereas small peripheral veins were readily sclerosed by such solutions, the slow, continuous infusion into a central vein, with its high blood flow, protected the intima of the vein from osmotically induced damage.

A great deal of experience has accumulated in pediatric patients with central venous *total parenteral nutrition* (TPN), and in selected groups of patients, spectacular clinical results, have been achieved judged by falls in mortality rates. In particular, gratifying results have been obtained in term infants born with surgically reparable major gastrointestinal anomalies and in post-term infants with chronic intractable diarrhea. Experience with these groups of patients has taught many valuable lessons, which will be summarized in the following paragraphs. However, the initial hope that central venous TPN would solve the problem of feeding the LBW and, especially, the VLBW infant has not been realized, not only because such infants are inherently at greater risk for catheter-related complications, especially sepsis, but also because they are much more labile metabolically, particularly with respect to glucose tolerance (see p. 83). A modification of central venous TPN has been developed for this group of infants in which smaller amounts of glucose are infused together with other nutrients through a peripheral vein.

The terms *total parenteral nutrition, hyperalimentation, total parenteral alimentation, intravenous hyperalimentation*, and *central* or *deep vein parenteral nutrition* have all been used to designate modifications of the technique initially described by Dudrick and co-workers. *Peripheral vein parenteral nutrition, peripheral total parenteral nutrition*, and *partial parenteral nutrition*, among others, have been used to describe the technique of providing nutrients by peripheral venous infusion. *Total* rather than *complete* parenteral nutrition is used to signify that the nutrient infusate does not necessarily supply all nutrient requirements. Total parenteral nutrition still seems to be the best term to describe the situation in which parenteral nutrients provide the sole (or total) nutritional support. In this discussion, this term will be further modified to designate the route of delivery—that is, central venous or peripheral venous delivery.

Since many of the problems of central venous TPN are shared by peripheral venous TPN, the two techniques will for the most part be treated together in the ensuing discussion. In passing, it should be mentioned that although the quantitative dimensions of the problem differ from the infant to the child and adult, the basic lessons that have been learned in the infant are applicable to the older child and the adult. Indeed, the case can be made that the infant is a much more sensitive indicator of the efficacy and the safety of parenteral nutrition than is the adult. It follows, therefore, that complications that occur in the infant are also likely to occur in the adult, although to a less severe degree.

### Indications and contraindications for parenteral nutrition

Parenteral nutrition is indicated for any patient who is unable to tolerate enteral feedings for a significant period of time. This significant period of time varies from patient to patient. For example, little convincing argument can be advanced for the necessity of using parenteral nutrients in the appropriate amounts for term newborn infants or for older infants in whom enteral nutrients must be withheld for only a few days owing to some acute illness that is likely to resolve. On the other hand, in the VLBW infant, limited endogenous energy stores make the need for parenteral nutrition much more intense, particularly in the face of uncertainty about the infant's ability to establish a completely adequate enteral intake.

Most pediatric patients requiring TPN are less than 1 year old, and most of these are less than 1 month old, but the various techniques are useful for any child or adult who cannot tolerate enteral intake for a significant period of time (e.g., owing to disorders such as fistulas and peritonitis, and inflammatory bowel disease, in selected patients).

In oliguric renal failure, a modification of TPN in which only the essential amino acids and high glucose concentrations (up to 70%) are given in a small volume of fluid has been shown to improve the multiple biochemical abnormalities and to reduce mortality.

There are few if any contraindications for the use of parenteral nutrition; however, since there are definite, potentially serious, short-term complications due to the technique, and since the long-term effects are not known with certainty, the technique should not be used indiscriminately. As has already been mentioned, there seems to be little indication for using parenteral nutrition during the first 24 to 48 hr of life unless the condition necessitating this therapy is expected to preclude enteral feedings for a protracted period of time, such as in infants with gastroschisis. Also, the use of central venous TPN for only a few days should be avoided if at all possible.

*Choice of route of delivery*
Once the decision has been made to institute parenteral nutrition, the route of therapy must be decided on. There are two general considerations that enter into this decision: (1) the nature of the disease process and, specifically, the expected time interval during which the enteral route will not likely be functional, and (2) the birth weight of the infant or, more specifically, the degree of glucose or fat intolerance that may be expected.

Term and post-term infants, and children and adults presenting with lesions that are likely to preclude any significant enteral intake for several weeks or more are prime candidates for central venous TPN, and in this group very gratifying results have been achieved. Barring significant ongoing stress, infants in this group can tolerate 120 Cal/kg/day, predominantly delivered as glucose, without significant (usually transient) hyperglycemia, provided the glucose intake is increased gradually (i.e., over a few days).

On the other hand, LBW infants with illnesses such as respiratory distress syndrome (RDS), in which only a few days of parenteral nutritional support are likely to be needed, are the prime candidates for peripheral venous parenteral nutrition. The most difficult problems arise with the LBW infant and, especially, the VLBW infant with disorders that require several weeks of parenteral nutrition. The glucose load needed to provide 120 Cal/kg/day far exceeds their expected glucose tolerance (see p. 83); further, they seem to show an inability to tolerate more than 1 to 2 g/kg/day of fat. Advantage can be taken of the fact that the caloric expenditure of these preterm infants can be reduced if assiduous attention is paid to maintaining a *thermoneutral environment*, defined as the ambient temperature at which oxygen consumption is minimal. Under these conditions, an intake of 60 Cal/kg/day from glucose plus 2.5 g/kg/day of amino acids, along with other nutrients (including a small amount of fat to cover essential fatty acid requirements) will promote positive nitrogen balance, and, depending on age, some weight gain, although less than is the case with the central venous TPN regimen.

The decision as to the route, however, boils down to an accurate forecast by an experienced clinician as to how long a given infant with a given disorder will be unable to take sufficient nutrients enterally. If anything, one should err on the conservative side in making this decision to avoid the all-too-common situation of having maintained an LBW or VLBW infant on peripheral venous infusions for a week or more showing a relatively unimpressive weight gain and all peripheral veins exhausted. Central venous infusion at the start of the course in such an infant would be preferable, but with the caveat that a caloric intake of 120 Cal/kg/day is unlikely to be achieved, although one higher than 60 Cal/kg/day could be achieved, if careful monitoring for hyperglycemia and glycosuria were carried out. Furthermore, the enteral route can often be used to provide some nutrients, and, if possible, this route should be used along with the parenteral route with due regard for the tolerance of the gut.

Finally, the choice of route of delivery should take account of the hospital's overall ability to deliver either type of parenteral nutrition. For example, if previous experience with TPN by central vein has been associated with a low incidence of both catheter-related and metabolic complications, there is little reason to with-

TABLE 20. Composition of a Suitable Parenteral Nutrient Infusate for Infants

| Component | Amount per Day |
| --- | --- |
| Crystalline amino acid mixture | 2.5 g/kg |
| Glucose[a] | 5–30 g/kg |
| Sodium (NaCl) | 3–4 mEq/kg |
| Potassium[b] | 2–3 mEq/kg |
| Calcium (Calcium gluconate) | 0.5–1.0 mEq/kg |
| Magnesium (MgSO$_4$) | 0.25 mEq/kg |
| Chloride | 3–4 mEq/kg |
| Phosphate [b] | 2 mM/kg |
| Zinc (ZnSO$_4$)[c] | 2.5–5.0 μM/kg |
| Copper (CuSO$_4$)[c] | 0.3 μM/kg |
| MVI[d] | 1–3 ml |
| Total volume | 120–150 ml/kg |

[a]Glucose can be reduced depending on the amount of intravenous fat emulsion used. The amount provided via the central vein should not exceed 15 g/kg/24 hr (see text) on the initial day of treatment. Concentrations greater that 10% usually cannot be given by a peripheral vein.

[b]Hyperphosphatemia often develops with phosphate intakes greater than 2 mM/kg/day; thus, if potassium intake of more than 2 mEq/kg/day is required, it should be provided as KCl.

[c]Suggested by Department of Foods and Nutrition, American Medical Association.

[d]U. S. Pharmaceutical, Tuckahoe, N.Y. This preparation (1 ml) contains adequate amounts of all required vitamins except folic acid, vitamin B$_{12}$ and vitamin K. Vitamin B$_{12}$ and vitamin K can be given by intramuscular injections.

hold this method of therapy. But if the reverse is true and central venous TPN is indicated, consideration should be given to transferring the patient to a more experienced institution, provided the underlying clinical situation is one that cannot be managed well by peripheral venous infusion.

*Composition of the nutrient infusate*

The composition of an infusate providing amino acids, a calorie source, electrolytes, minerals, trace metals, and vitamins is shown in Table 20. Solutions for either central venous or peripheral venous infusion vary in their glucose content, but they are otherwise similar.

At present, four different commercially available crystalline amino-acid solutions are available; formerly, hydrolysates of either fibrin or casein were used as nitrogen sources. Both types of nitrogen sources provide most essential as well as nonessential amino acids, although none of the crystalline mixtures or the hydrolysates contain a pattern of amino acids that could be considered ideal in the sense of producing a plasma amino-acid pattern resembling the normal postprandial concentrations of amino acids seen after oral feedings of normal infants.

Furthermore, no available mixture contains cystine or more than a trace of tyrosine, amino acids that are highly insoluble but probably essential for the premature and term infant. A cysteine : HCl additive is available, but its efficacy in meeting the cystine requirement is uncertain.

In the typical infant, an amino acid intake of 2.5 g/kg/day should result in a daily nitrogen retention of about 0.2 g/kg/day and a steady-state weight gain of about 13 g/kg/day, values comparable to those seen in infants fed enterally.

Glucose, used alone or with fat emulsions (see the following paragraphs), is the most commonly used caloric source. Provision of a daily caloric intake of approximately 120 Cal/kg/day is necessary to assure optimal growth in the term and post-term infant. In general, glucose intakes greater than 15 g/kg/day are not tolerated on the first day of therapy, but intake can usually be increased in increments of 5 g/kg/day until the desired level is achieved.

Using the peripheral route in LBW and VLBW infants, a fluid volume of 150 ml/kg/day providing 10% glucose will provide about 60 Cal/kg/day. Larger volumes can sometimes be used, but these cannot be recommended routinely since much depends on the individual infant's tolerance.

### Use of intravenous fat emulsions

Intravenous fat emulsions serve two general purposes in the parenteral nutritional regimen: (1) to prevent *essential fatty acid* (EFA) deficiency, and (2) to provide a source of calories in an iso-osmotic vehicle.

The currently available preparations Intralipid and Liposyn consist of soybean or safflower oil emulsions, respectively, and a phosphatide emulsifier. The emulsion itself exerts no osmotic effect. Glycerol (a carbohydrate) is added to make the solution iso-osmotic (300 mOsm/L). Such emulsions at 10 percent concentration would provide 100 g/L (90 Cal/100 ml) from fat plus 20 Cal/100 ml (from glycerol), giving a total of 110 Cal/100 ml or 1.1 Cal/ml.

It is clear that chemical EFA deficiency will develop promptly in infants, children, and adults in whom successful anabolism is initiated by the provision of all nutrients needed for growth, except EFA. Clinical signs of EFA deficiency, on the other hand, are uncommon, erratic in appearance, and seem generally confined to long-standing EFA-deficient patients. The amount of a fat emulsion assumed to prevent EFA deficiency is equivalent to about 4 percent of the total caloric intake or less than 1 g/kg/day of fat. This amount can be given daily, although somewhat more can be given on a twice weekly schedule.

The use of fat emulsions as a caloric source poses many more uncertainties than using them to meet EFA requirements since 2 to 3 g/kg/day or more would be required to make a significant impact on total caloric intake. The uncertainties revolve around such incompletely resolved problems as tolerance as a function of gestational age, interference with pulmonary function, competition of free fatty acids with bilirubin or albumin, nonequivalence of a fat calorie with a carbohydrate calorie in inducing nitrogen retention, interference with phagocytic function, and so forth.

Given the limited information available, it is difficult to make specific recommendations about the use of intravenous fat emulsions in pediatric patients—particularly in premature infants. In general, a dose of 1 g/kg/day is probably safe for almost all infants, provided it is administered slowly. Larger doses should be used with caution, particularly in patients with underlying pulmonary disease or hyperbilirubinemia. Use of fat emulsions in amounts greater than those needed to meet the EFA requirements probably should be avoided in any infant with a plasma bilirubin above 8 to 10 mg/100 ml.

*Techniques of infusion*
Figure 34 shows the delivery system used for central venous TPN. A silicone rubber (Silastic) catheter is threaded into the internal jugular vein until its tip, verified radiographically, lies in the superior vena cava just above the right atrium. The other end of the catheter is directed through a skin tunnel to exit on the parietal scalp where the occlusive dressings are more readily accessible for changing. The neck incision is then closed. All fluids are mixed in a laminar flow hood since they are excellent media for bacteria and especially for candida. All fluids are pumped at a specified rate; a 0.22 μ membrane filter serves as an additional precaution in filtering bacteria and particulate matter. One should change the dressings three times a week, observing strict aseptic principles. It is generally believed that lapses in the technique of changing dressings are the leading contributor to sepsis, followed by contamination of infusates either in their manufacture or by violating the system once it is in place, by blood drawing or administration of

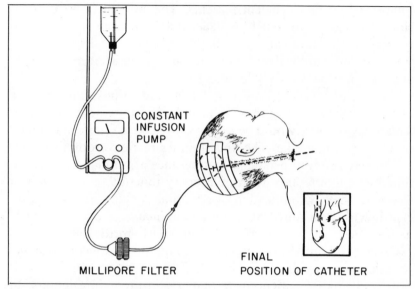

FIGURE 34. Technique of insertion of the catheter into the internal jugular vein and its location in the superior vena cava.

drugs or other solutions through the central line. With strict adherence to these measures for catheter care as well as the preparation of solutions aseptically, the rate of sepsis should be less than 6 percent, even in the smallest of infants.

When fat emulsions are to be given, the delivery system must be modified, since the glucose-amino acid solution, when directly mixed with fat, causes the emulsion to be destabilized. Thus, fat emulsions must be infused by piggybacking the fat emulsion using a Y connector to join it with the glucose-amino acid mixture near the entrance to the catheter. Generally, it is necessary to use separate infusion pumps for the lipid emulsion and the glucose-amino acid mixture.

Nutrient mixtures for peripheral venous TPN are usually infused into one of the superficial veins of the dorsal aspect of either the hand or foot or into one of the superficial veins of the scalp. In most cases, scalp vein needles are used. Use of a 25-gauge scalp vein needle with both a short bevel and a short length makes insertion technically easier. In addition, this needle can be secured more easily and without much tape, thereby decreasing the likelihood of undetected extravasation. A 22-gauge Medicut needle that allows percutaneous placement of a Silastic catheter can also be used. The experience and expertise of the team responsible for establishing and maintaining the infusion should determine the

TABLE 21. Metabolic Complications of Total Parenteral Nutrition and Their Most Common Causes

| Metabolic Disorder | Usual Cause |
|---|---|
| Disorders related to metabolic capacity of patient | |
| Hyperglycemia | Excessive intake of glucose (either excessive concentration of increased infusion rate). Change in metabolic state (e.g., sepsis, surgical stress) |
| Hypoglycemia | Sudden cessation of infusion |
| Azotemia | Excessive nitrogen intake |
| Electrolyte disorders | Excessive or inadequate intake |
| Mineral (major and trace) disorders | Excessive or inadequate intake |
| Vitamin disorders | Excessive or inadequate intake |
| Essential fatty acid deficiency | Failure to provide essential fatty acids |
| Disorders related to infustate components | |
| Acid-base disorders (hyperchloremic metabolic acidosis) | Use of hydrochloride salts of cationic amino acids |
| Hyperammonemia | Inadequate arginine intake |
| Abnormal plasma aminograms | Amino acid pattern of nitrogen source |
| Hepatic disorders | Unknown |

specific method used. Caution in placement of the scalp vein needle or the Medicut catheter as well as subsequent meticulous care of the site will minimize the complications of this general method of nutrient delivery.

*Metabolic complications*

Two general types of metabolic complications have been associated with parenteral nutrition: (1) those resulting from the patient's limited metabolic capacity for the various components of the nutrient infusate, and (2) those related to the inherent properties of the infusate itself (Table 21). Of complications in the first group, carbohydrate intolerance is the most frequently encountered. While most patients can easily tolerate glucose in the amount of 10 to 15 g/kg/day, some are intolerant to doses as small as 5 g/kg/day; this is particularly those with ongoing stress (surgery, sepsis, and so forth) and, of course, the LBW and, especially, the VLBW infant. Electrolyte and mineral disorders usually are due to the provision of too much or too little of these substances in relation to increased urinary losses secondary to osmotic diuresis or to other abnormal losses.

The metabolic complications due to inherent properties of the infusate—usually the amino acid mixtures—are more troublesome. No currently available amino acid mixture results in a completely normal plasma amino acid pattern. Concern for the effects of such abnormalities is based principally on the long-recognized association between mental retardation and various, abnormal plasma-amino acid concentrations in patients with various inborn errors of metabolism (e.g., phenylketonuria, maple syrup urine disease, and so forth). Furthermore, no currently available amino acid mixture contains sufficient amounts of the poorly soluble amino acids, cystine and tyrosine. The generally abnormal plasma amino acid patterns plus the lack of these two essential amino acids may result in a decreased efficacy of current TPN practices, and, in fact, may explain the observation that no one amino acid solution can be shown to be superior to any other, including the hydrolysates, when they are assessed by such relatively crude measures as nitrogen balance or weight gain.

## Infusion-related complications
Infusion-related complications of central venous TPN include thrombosis and catheter displacement and infection. All unfortunately occur from time to time with long-term catheterization. Their occurrence can be reduced to an acceptable level by careful adherence to established rules for catheter insertion and care. This category of complications occurring with peripheral venous TPN includes skin and subcutaneous sloughs secondary to the infiltration of the hypertonic infusate. If infection occurs with peripheral venous delivery, it is usually due to a contaminated infusate; whereas, with central venous delivery it is usually secondary to contamination of the catheter exit site.

## Requirements for successful parenteral nutrition
Successful parenteral nutrition requires constant vigilance and dedicated, knowledgeable personnel as well as specialized facilities. Only in this way can complications be minimized and the benefits of this form of nutritional management be maximized.

For good success, experience has shown that this form of therapy should be carried out by a trained parenteral nutrition team.

The key member of such a team should be a physician who is fully acquainted with nutritional biochemistry and who assumes responsibility for the day-to-day details of the parenteral nutrition program as well as for educating junior and senior staff in this relatively new area of knowledge. Another member of the team should be the TPN nurse who works exclusively with parenteral nutrition or with the hospital's nutritional support team. This nurse's duties may be primarily educational, especially if the patients requiring parenteral nutrition are scattered in several units throughout the hospital. Alternatively, the nurse may be responsible for all specialized aspects of the care of the patient, the most important being the changing of the central venous dressings on a triweekly basis. One well-trained person who meticulously performs this task is a guarantee against a high sepsis rate.

Another requirement for a successful TPN team is a flexible system for mixing parenteral infusates. The increasingly common practice of mixing stock solutions routinely and storing them until used, while obviously more convenient and economical, cannot be recommended for pediatric patients since metabolic instability in the infant often requires that TPN fluids be tailor-made to his needs as they are defined by serial monitoring. Special facilities are needed for aseptic preparation of large-volume parenteral fluid preparations. Ideally, a pharmacist trained in aseptic mixing techniques should be assigned full-time or part-time to the TPN team. In general, infusates for central venous TPN should be prepared every 2 to 3 days. Unused solutions should be discarded after this time.

Only in patients with demonstrated long-term metabolic stability can infusates be expected to be similar from day to day. In these cases, it may be possible to store the solutions for several days, perhaps even a week or so. Since the stability of the multiple-vitamin preparation that is added to the solution is unknown, it is probably best to add this preparation under aseptic conditions on the day of infusion.

Successful parenteral nutrition requires a responsive microchemical laboratory for chemical monitoring. Routine microbiologic cultures of the nutrient infusate or routine blood cultures, as are often suggested, are unnecessary after one is convinced that the pharmacist and the TPN nurse are carrying out their respective

TABLE 22. Variables to be Monitored During Intravenous Nutrition, with Suggested Frequency of Monitoring

| Variables | Suggested Frequency* | |
| | Initial Period | Later Period |
| --- | --- | --- |
| Growth variables | | |
|   Weight | Daily | Daily |
|   Length | Weekly | Weekly |
|   Head circumference | Weekly | Weekly |
| Metabolic variables | | |
|   Blood measurements | | |
|     Plasma electrolytes | 3–4 times weekly | Weekly |
|     Blood urea nitrogen | 3–4 times weekly | Weekly |
|     Plasma Ca, Mg, P | 2 times weekly | Weekly |
|     Acid-base status | 3–4 times weekly | Weekly |
|     Serum protein (PEP or albumin) | Weekly | Weekly |
|     Liver function studies | Weekly | Weekly |
|     Hemoglobin | 2 times weekly | 2 times weekly |
|   Urine glucose | 4–6 times daily | 2 times daily |
| Prevention and detection of infection | | |
|   Clinical observations (activity, temperature, and so forth) | Daily | Daily |
|   White blood cell count and differential | As indicated | As indicated |
| Cultures | As indicated | As indicated |

*The initial period is that period in which a full glocose intake is being achieved; the later period is that time when the patient has achieved a steady metabolic state. In the presence of metabolic instability, the more intensive monitoring suggested for the initial period should be followed.

tasks with due regard for preventing sepsis. However, a responsive microbiologic laboratory must be available in suspected cases of sepsis. One routine maneuver that is helpful, both in assessing the adequacy of catheter care as well as in determining the precise organism involved should an infection occur, is a culture of the skin at the catheter site that is obtained at the time of each dressing change.

## Monitoring parenteral nutrition
Careful monitoring of the patient requiring parenteral nutrition is necessary to detect complications as well as to assess the clinical results. Both of these tasks require personnel who are familiar with the many intricacies of parenteral nutrition, including the

special apparatus required for the delivery system (e.g., the many varieties of constant infusion pumps).

A suggested schedule for biochemical monitoring is shown in Table 22. Adherence to this schedule will usually allow detection of controllable metabolic complications in sufficient time to permit their correction by altering the composition of the infusate. Routine monitoring of blood glucose concentration is not required if the urine is checked regularly (at least four times daily) for the presence of glucose; more frequently monitoring is necessary during the first few days after starting technique. As long as the urine is free of glucose, it is safe to assume that the blood glucose concentration is not unreasonably high. While Dextrostix determinations are not sufficiently accurate to detect severe hyperglycemia, they are useful for detecting hypoglycemia, which may occur with sudden cessation of the infusion due to delivery malfunction.

Blood ammonia is difficult to measure in many hospitals. A slight hyperammonemia is often seen in TPN. A vivid experience taught the author that knowledge of the blood ammonia concentration may be very informative in patients who show sudden neurologic deterioration in the face of normal values for all the biochemical measures shown in Table 22. In four such patients, severe hyperammonemia, ultimately traceable to arginine deficiency in an early composition of an amino acid solution was discovered. This no longer appears to be a problem with current solutions. While plasma amino acid concentrations during TPN provide useful research information, they are expensive, difficult to obtain, and of questionable routine clinical value.

A very troublesome area concerns the monitoring of intravenous fat infusions. Direct observation of the plasma turbidity and its measurement by nephelometry have been suggested as a means of detecting overt lipemia. However, neither procedure is useful for detecting elevated concentrations of free fatty acids and, in fact, may not even reliably predict plasma triglycerides. Thus, truly reliable monitoring of fat emulsions requires the actual chemical determination of plasma triglyceride, cholesterol, and free fatty acid concentrations—determinations that are not commonly available in most institutions, particularly on microsamples. Further progress in this area is needed for the safe use of intravenous fat emulsions.

# Glossary

ACID. A substance capable of donating a hydrogen ion or proton ($Ha \longrightarrow H^+ \ a^-$).

ACIDEMIA. An abnormality in blood characterized by a low blood pH.

ACIDOSIS. An abnormal physiologic process characterized by gain of acid or loss of base from the extracellular fluid.

ALKALEMIA. An abnormality in blood characterized by a high blood pH.

ALKALOSIS. An abnormal physiologic process characterized by gain of base or loss of acid from the extracellular fluid.

ANION. An ion that bears a negative charge.

ANION GAP. A computation, represented as either plasma ($[Na^+]$) − ($[Cl^-] + [HCO_3^-]$) or plasma ($[Na^+] + [K^+]$) − ($[Cl^-] + [HCO_3^-]$) that gives an approximate measure of the sum of the organic anions, phosphate, and sulfate in plasma.

ANTIDIURETIC HORMONE (ADH). A hormone derived from the posterior pituitary gland that stimulates the renal reabsorption of water.

BALANCE PRINCIPLE. The balance of any substance is equal to the intake by all routes minus the output by all routes. The balance may be zero (intake = output), positive (intake > output), or negative (intake < output).

BASE. Any substance capable of accepting a hydrogen ion ($a^- + H^+ \longrightarrow Ha$); a conjugate base is the base dissociated from a given acid ($a^-$ is the conjugate of Ha).

BASE DEFICIT OR BASE EXCESS. A measure of the change in the concentration of all conjugate bases in 1 L of a given sample of whole blood from the expected normal value for conjugate bases when the blood has a normal acid-base status; base deficit (BD) or base excess (BE) = observed buffer base − normal buffer base. The dimensions are mEq/L of whole blood.

BUFFER BASE. The sum of the concentration of all conjugate bases in 1 L of whole blood; blood buffer base (BB) = $[HCO_3^-] + [\,Buf^-\,]$. The dimensions are mEq/L of whole blood.

BUFFER PAIR. A weak acid and its conjugate base that when present in a solution minimize change in pH on addition of acid or base.

CALORIC EXPENDITURE. The energy expenditure of the body measured as kcal or Cal per day; unless otherwise specified, the caloric expenditure includes the basal energy expenditure plus the energy expended for activity.

CATION. An ion that bears a positive charge.

COMPENSATION. A secondary physiologic process whereby the pH deviation produced by a primary disturbance in blood acid-base status is ameliorated; in metabolic disorders, compensation is respiratory; whereas, in respiratory disorders compensation is renal.

CONJUGATE BASE. See Base.

DEFICITS OF WATER OR ELECTROLYTES. Refers to previously incurred losses of water or electrolyte that have occurred through negative balances of these substances as the result of disease; such previously incurred negative balances lead to a fall, or deficit, of body stores of water or specific electrolytes.

DEHYDRATION. A rather vague term used by some authors to denote loss of body water as well as electrolyte and by others to imply loss of body water alone. In this book, dehydration is used in the latter context.

DENOMINATOR TERM. Refers to the denominator of the ratio of the Henderson-Hasselbalch equation; the denominator can be depicted as $CO_{2(d)} + H_2CO_3$. Alternatively, because of Henry's law, the denominator may be expressed as $PCO_2 \times S$ or $PCO_2 \times 0.03$. The dimensions of the denominator term are millimoles per liter.

ELECTROLYTES. Any substance that when dissolved in water dissociates into ions, thus rendering the solution capable of conducting electricity; the dimensions of electrolytes are usually expressed in milliequivalents per liter (mEq/L).

EXTRACELLULAR FLUID (ECF). That compartment of the total body water that is excluded from cells. The ECF includes the interstitial fluid (ISF) and the plasma volume (PV).

"GAMBLEGRAM. "A diagrammatic representation of the ionic content of body fluids whereby the milliequivalents contributed by the cations are plotted in one column and those contributed by the anions in another. The two columns must be equal because of the law of electroneutrality.

GLOMERULAR FILTRATION. The process by which renal arterial blood is filtered by the glomeruli of the kidney to produce a protein-free ultrafiltrate, which is then acted on selectively by the renal tubules.

HENDERSON-HASSELBALCH EQUATION. A general quantitative equation that relates pH to the concentrations of weak acid and conjugate base in a buffer solution. In its most general form, the equation states that

$$pH = pK' + \log \frac{\text{conjugate base}}{\text{weak acid}}$$

where pK′ is a constant specific for the particular buffer pair.

HENRY'S LAW. A gas law that states that the amount of gas dissolved in a liquid is proportional (through the solubility coefficient) to the pressure of the gas in the gas phase. For $CO_2$: $PCO_2 \times S = CO_{2(d)} + H_2CO_3$. The dimensions of $PCO_2$ are mm Hg; those of $S$ are mM/L/mm Hg; and those of $CO_{2(d)} + H_2CO_3$ are mM/L.

HYPER- AND HYPOBASEMIA. Values for plasma bicarbonate concentration or whole blood buffer base excess that are greater or less than normal, respectively.

HYPER- AND HYPOCAPNIA (OR -CARBIA). Values for alveolar (and, hence, arterial) $PCO_2$ that are greater or less than normal, respectively.

HYPER- AND HYPOCHLOREMIA. Values for plasma chloride concentration significantly above or below normal, respectively.

HYPER- AND HYPOKALEMIA. Values for plasma potassium concentration significantly above or below normal, respectively.

HYPER- AND HYPONATREMIA. Values for plasma sodium concentration significantly above or below normal, respectively.

HYPER- AND HYPO-OSMOTIC. Solutions that are higher or lower as to normal osmolarity, respectively. These terms are used interchangeably with hyper- and hypotonic.

HYPER- AND HYPOTONIC. Solutions that cause erythrocytes to shrink or swell, respectively; such solutions contain more or less, respectively, of osmotically active (nonpermeable) solutes. These terms are used interchangeably with hyper- and hypo-osmotic.

INTERSTITIAL FLUID (ISF). A subcompartment of the extracellular fluid that includes all ECF except that present in blood volume.

INTRACELLULAR FLUID (ICF). A compartment of the body water that includes all water within the cells of all tissues.

ION. Any electrically charged particle.

ISO-OSMOTIC. A solution that contains 280 mOsm/L of nonpenetrating solute. This term is interchangeable with isotonic.

ISOTONIC. A solution that causes neither swelling nor shrinking of the erythrocyte. This corresponds to an osmolarity of 280 mOsm/L and is therefore interchangeable with iso-osmotic.

MAINTENANCE REQUIREMENTS OR MAINTENANCE THERAPY. The

amount of water and electrolyte necessary to maintain the organism in zero balance for these substances. Normal maintenance requirements are those required for the usual ongoing processes of insensible water loss, urine formation, sweating, and losses of water in the stool. Abnormal maintenance requirements include replacement of losses sustained through normal routes in abnormal amounts or through abnormal routes.

METABOLIC ACIDOSIS. An abnormal physiologic state due to gain of strong acid or loss of bicarbonate from the ECF.

METABOLIC ALKALOSIS. An abnormal physiologic state due to gain of strong base or gain of bicarbonate by the ECF.

MILLIEQUIVALENT (mEq). A measure of the electrical charge contributed by an ion in terms of its ability to combine with ions of the opposite charge.

$$1 \text{ mEq of an ion} = \frac{\text{atomic or ionic weight (in mg)}}{\text{valence of the ion}}$$

$$\text{For example,} \quad 1 \text{ mEq of Ca}^{++} = \frac{40 \text{ mg}}{2} = 20 \text{ mg}$$

$$1 \text{ mEq of Na}^{+} - \frac{23 \text{ mg}}{1} = 23 \text{ mg}$$

MILLIMOL (mM). The molecular weight of a substance (ion or molecule) in milligrams; for example,

1 mM of dextrose $(C_6H_{12}O_6)$ = 72 + 12 + 96 = 180 mg
1 mM of NaCl = 23 + 35.5 = 58.5 mg

MILLIOSMOL (mOsm). A measure of the osmotic contribution of a solute; this property is independent of the size or charge of solute; mOsm contributed by a solute equals mM of solute times $n$ where $n$ is the number of particles produced by dissociation. Thus, 1 mM $CaCl_2$ produces 3 mOsm since $n$ is 3 (one $Ca^{++}$ and 2 $Cl^-$). For nondissociating solutes (e.g. dextrose) $n$ is 1.

NET ACID EXCRETION (NAE). The daily urinary excretion (mEq/day) of acid or base, defined as the sum of ammonium plus titratable acid minus bicarbonate.

NONBICARBONATE BUFFERS. A class of buffers that includes all buffers in body fluids except the bicarbonate system. In blood, the principal nonbicarbonate buffers are hemoglobin and oxyhemoglobin, and smaller contributions are made by plasma proteins and inorganic and organic phosphates. The symbols used for the nonbicarbonate buffers are HBuf for all weak acids and Buf$^-$ for all conjugate bases.

NONPENETRATING SOLUTE. Solutes that permeate poorly or do not permeate cell membranes, such as $Na^+$ or $Cl^-$. Freely permeating solutes in body fluids are urea and $CO_{2(d)}$.

NUMERATOR TERM. Refers to the numerator term in the ratio of the Henderson-Hasselbalch equation—i.e., the bicarbonate concentration of the plasma.

OSMOLARITY. The total osmotic contribution by all solutes per liter of solution; i.e., mOsm/L. In physiology, effective osmolarity refers to mOsm contributed by nonpenetrating solutes ($Na^+$, $Cl^-$, and so forth); total osmolarity includes penetrating solutes (urea, and so forth) as well.

$PCO_2$. The partial pressure of carbon dioxide in alveolar gas. Since alveolar gas and arterial blood are in equilibrium, one can speak of arterial $PCO_2$, which is the pressure of $CO_2$ in alveolar air necessary to give observed result for denominator term (see Henry's law). The dimensions of $PCO_2$ are mm Hg.

pH. A measure of the free hydrogen ion ($H^+$) concentration of a solution; $pH = \dfrac{1}{\log H^+}$ . Thus, a pH of 7.0 is equal to 0.0000001 mole of $H^+$ per liter, while a pH of 1.0 is 0.1 mole of $H^+$ per liter. Thus, the higher the pH the lower the $H^+$.

pK'. A constant in the Henderson-Hasselbalch equation related to the dissociation constant of the weak acid of the buffer pair. For the bicarbonate buffer system in normal plasma, a pK' has a value of 6.10.

PLASMA VOLUME (PV). A subcompartment of the extracellular fluid consisting of that part of the ECF within the capillary membrane.

PLASMA WATER CONCENTRATION. The amount of water in one liter of plasma. Normal plasma contains 93% water; i.e., plasma water concentration is 0.93 L of water per liter of plasma.

PREFORMED WATER. Water released from cells when cells are catabolized, as in wasting disease.

PRERENAL AZOTEMIA. Elevation of BUN and plasma creatinine concentration occurring as the result of a reduction in renal circulation and glomerular filtration rate; prerenal azotemia is to be differentiated from renal azotemia where glomerular filtration is reduced because of intrinsic glomerular disease.

R FRACTION. Residual fraction. See Anion gap.

RESPIRATORY ACIDOSIS. An abnormal physiologic state characterized by a primary decrease in alveolar ventilation due to some disease or disorder of the respiratory system.

RESPIRATORY ALKALOSIS. An abnormal physiologic state characterized by a primary increase in alveolar ventilation due to some disease or disorder of the respiratory system.

$S$. The solubility coefficient of $CO_2$ in normal plasma at normal body temperature; the value for $S$ is 0.03 mM/L/mm Hg.

SOLUTE. Any substance dissolved in a solvent that thereby forms a solution.

TITRATABLE ACID (TA). The amount of urinary $H^+$ excretion that is bound to buffers determined by titration of urine from its actual pH to pH 7.40.

TOTAL BODY WATER (TBW). All water in the body, regardless of whether it is in the intracellular or the extracellular compartment.

TOTAL PARENTERAL NUTRITION (TPN). The provision of all nutrients by the central or peripheral venous route. TPN is to be differentiated from complete parenteral nutrition, which assumes that the intake is nutritionally complete. Because of lack of knowledge, the latter may not be possible at this time.

TUBULAR (RENAL) REABSORPTION. Any process by which the renal tubular cells transport substances from tubular urine into peritubular plasma and, hence, into the renal venous blood.

TUBULAR (RENAL) SECRETION. Any process by which renal tubular cells transport substances from peritubular plasma into tubular urine.

TUBULAR (RENAL) URINE. Fluid within the lumen of the renal tubules that is acted on by tubular reabsorption of tubular secretion to produce the final (bladder) urine.

UNDETERMINED ANION (UA). That fraction of the plasma anions that is not ordinarily determined in routine clinical chemistry laboratories. It is the difference between the determined cations ($Na^+$, $K^+$, $Ca^{++}$, $Mg^{++}$) and the usually determined anions ($Cl^-$, $HCO_3^-$, and proteinate). UA contains inorganic phosphate, inorganic sulfate, and small contributions from a number of organic anions.

WATER OF OXIDATION. Water produced in oxidation of foodstuffs by cells. Normally, this amounts to about 10 ml of water per 100 Calories expended.

# Index

# Index